Virtual Clinical Excursions—Medical-Surgical

for

Christensen and Kockrow:
Adult Health Nursing
5th Edition

Virtual Clinical Excursions—Medical-Surgical

for

Christensen and Kockrow:
Adult Health Nursing
5th Edition

prepared by

Kim D. Cooper, RN, MSN
Ivy Tech Community College
Terre Haute, Indiana

software developed by

Wolfsong Informatics, LLC
Tucson, Arizona

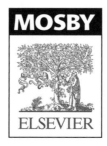

MOSBY

ELSEVIER

11830 Westline Industrial Dr.
St. Louis, Missouri 63146

VIRTUAL CLINICAL EXCURSIONS—MEDICAL-SURGICAL FOR
CHRISTENSEN AND KOCKROW:
ADULT HEALTH NURSING
5TH EDITION

ISBN-13: 978-0-323-04338-0
ISBN-10: 0-323-04338-0

Copyright © 2007 by Mosby, Inc., an affiliate of Elsevier Inc.

Although for mechanical reasons all pages of this publication are perforated, only those pages
imprinted with a Mosby, Inc., an affiliate of Elsevier Inc. copyright notice are intended for removal.

Notice

Knowledge and best practice in this field are constantly changing. As new research and experience
broaden our knowledge, changes in practice, treatment and drug therapy may become necessary or
appropriate. Readers are advised to check the most current information provided (i) on procedures
featured or (ii) by the manufacturer of each product to be administered, to verify the recommended
dose or formula, the method and duration of administration, and contraindications. It is the
responsibility of the practitioner, relying on their own experience and knowledge of the patient, to
make diagnoses, to determine dosages and the best treatment for each individual patient, and to
take all appropriate safety precautions. To the fullest extent of the law, neither the Publisher nor
the Authors assumes any liability for any injury and/or damage to persons or property arising out
or related to any use of the material contained in this book.

ISBN-13: 978-0-323-04338-0
ISBN-10: 0-323-04338-0

Executive Editor: *Tom Wilhelm*
Managing Editor: *Jeff Downing*
Associate Developmental Editor: *Tiffany Trautwein*
Project Manager: *Joy Moore*

Printed in the United States of America

Last digit is the print number: 9 8 7 6 5 4 3 2 1

*Workbook
prepared by*

Kim D. Cooper, RN, MSN
Ivy Tech Community College
Terre Haute, Indiana

Textbook

Barbara Lauritsen Christensen RN, MS
Nurse Educator
Mid-Plains Community College
North Platte, Nebraska

Elaine Oden Kockrow, RN, MS
Formerly, Nurse Educator
Mid-Plains Community College
North Platte, Nebraska

Contents

Table of Contents
Christensen and Kockrow:
Adult Health Nursing, 5th Edition

Getting Started

GETTING SET UP

■ **MINIMUM SYSTEM REQUIREMENTS**

WINDOWS™

Windows XP, 2000, 98, ME, NT 4.0 (Recommend Windows XP/2000)
Pentium® III processor (or equivalent) @ 600 MHz (Recommend 800 MHz or better)
128 MB of RAM (Recommend 256 MB or more)
800 x 600 screen size (Recommend 1024 x 768)
Thousands of colors
12x CD-ROM drive
Soundblaster 16 soundcard compatibility
Stereo speakers or headphones

Note: Virtual Clinical Excursion—Medical-Surgical for Windows will require a minimal
amount of disk space to install icons and required dll files for Windows 98/ME.

MACINTOSH®

MAC OS X (10.2 or higher)
Apple Power PC G3 @ 500 MHz or better
128 MB of RAM (Recommend 256 MB or more)
800 x 600 screen size (Recommend 1024 x 768)
Thousands of colors
12x CD-ROM drive
Stereo speakers or headphones

■ INSTALLATION INSTRUCTIONS

WINDOWS

1. Insert the *Virtual Clinical Excursion—Medical-Surgical* CD-ROM.
2. Inserting the CD should automatically bring up the setup screen if the current product is not already installed.
   a. If the setup screen does not appear automatically (and *Virtual Clinical Excursion—Medical-Surgical* has not been installed already), navigate to the "My Computer" icon on your desktop or in your Start menu.
   b. Double-click on your CD-ROM drive.
   c. If installation does not start at this point:
      (1) Click the **Start** icon on the task bar and select the **Run** option.
      (2) Type d:\setup.exe (where "d:\" is your CD-ROM drive) and press **OK**.
      (3) Follow the onscreen instructions for installation.
3. Follow the onscreen instructions during the setup process.

MACINTOSH

1. Insert the *Virtual Clinical Excursion—Medical-Surgical* CD in the CD-ROM drive. The disk icon will appear on your desktop.

2. Double-click on the disk icon.

3. Double-click on the MEDICAL-SURGICAL_MAC run file.

NOTE: *Virtual Clinical Excursion—Medical-Surgical* for Macintosh does not have an installation setup and can only be run directly from the CD.

■ HOW TO USE VIRTUAL CLINICAL EXCURSIONS—MEDICAL-SURGICAL

WINDOWS

1. Double-click on the *Virtual Clinical Excursion—Medical-Surgical* icon located on your desktop.
2. Or navigate to the program via the Windows Start menu.

NOTE: Windows 98/ME will require you to restart your computer before running the *Virtual Clinical Excursion—Medical-Surgical* program.

MACINTOSH

1. Insert the *Virtual Clinical Excursion—Medical-Surgical* CD in the CD-ROM drive. The disk icon will appear on your desktop.

2. Double-click on the disk icon.

3. Double-click on the MEDICAL-SURGICAL_MAC run file.

■ SCREEN SETTINGS

For best results, your computer monitor resolution should be set at a minimum of 800 x 600. The number of colors displayed should be set to "thousands or higher" (High Color or 16 bit) or "millions of colors" (True Color or 24 bit).

Windows™

1. From the **Start** menu, select **Control Panel** (on some systems, you will first go to **Settings**, then to **Control Panel**).
2. Double-click on the **Display** icon.
3. Click on the **Settings** tab.
4. Under **Screen area** use the slider bar to select **800 by 600 pixels**.
5. Access the **Colors** drop-down menu by clicking on the down arrow.
6. Select **High Color (16 bit)** or **True Color (24 bit)**.
7. Click on **OK**.
8. You may be asked to verify the setting changes. Click **Yes**.
9. You may be asked to restart your computer to accept the changes. Click **Yes**.

Macintosh®

1. Select the **Monitors** control panel.
2. Select **800 x 600** (or similar) from the **Resolution** area.
3. Select **Thousands** or **Millions** from the **Color Depth** area.

■ WEB BROWSERS

Supported web browsers include Microsoft Internet Explorer (IE) version 6.0 or higher, Netscape version 7.1 or higher, and Mozilla version 1.4 or higher.

If you use America Online (AOL) for web access, you will need AOL version 4.0 or higher and IE 5.0 or higher. Do not use earlier versions of AOL with earlier versions of IE, because you will have difficulty accessing many features.

For best results with AOL:
- Connect to the Internet using AOL version 4.0 or higher.
- Open a private chat within AOL (this allows the AOL client to remain open, without asking whether you wish to disconnect while minimized).
- Minimize AOL.
- Launch a recommended browser.

■ TECHNICAL SUPPORT

Technical support for this product is available between 7:30 a.m. and 7 p.m. CST, Monday through Friday. Before calling, be sure that your computer meets the minimum system requirements to run this software. Inside the United States and Canada, call 1-800-692-9010. Outside North America, call 314-872-8370. You may also fax your questions to 314-523-4932 or contact Technical Support through e-mail: technical.support@elsevier.com.

Trademarks: Windows, Macintosh, Pentium, and America Online are registered trademarks.

ACCESSING *Virtual Clinical Excursions—Medical-Surgical*
FROM EVOLVE

The product you have purchased is part of the Evolve family of online courses and learning resources. Please read the following information completely to get started.

To access your instructor's course on Evolve:

Your instructor will provide you with the username and password needed to access their specific course on the Evolve Learning System. Once you have received this information, please follow these instructions:

1. Go to the Evolve student page (http://evolve.elsevier.com/student)

2. Enter your username and password in the **Login to My Evolve** area and click the **Login** button.

3. You will be taken to your personalized **My Evolve** page where the course will be listed in the **My Courses** module.

TECHNICAL REQUIREMENTS

To use an Evolve course, you will need access to a computer that is connected to the Internet and equipped with web browser software that supports frames. For optimal performance, it is recommended that you have speakers and use a high-speed Internet connection. However, slower dial-up modems (56 K minimum) are acceptable.

Whichever browser you use, the browser preferences must be set to enable cookies and Java/JavaScript and the cache must be set to reload every time.

Enable Cookies

Browser	Steps
Internet Explorer (IE) 6.0 or higher	1. Select **Tools**. 2. Select **Internet Options**. 3. Select **Privacy** tab. 4. Use the slider (slide down) to **Accept All Cookies**. 5. Click **OK**. -OR- 4. Click the **Advanced** button. 5. Click the check box next to **Override Automatic Cookie Handling**. 6. Click the **Accept** buttons under **First-party Cookies** and **Third-party Cookies**. 7. Click **OK**.
Netscape 7.1 or higher	1. Select **Edit**. 2. Select **Preferences**. 3. Select **Privacy & Security**. 4. Select **Cookies**. 5. Select **Enable All Cookies**.
Mozilla 1.4 or higher	1. Select **Tools**. 2. Select **Privacy**. 3. Expand the **Cookies** section and check the following box: Allow sites to set cookies.

Enable Java

Browser	Steps
Internet Explorer (IE) 6.0 or higher	1. Select **Tools → Internet Options**. 2. Select **Advanced** tab. 3. Scroll down the list until you see the **Java (Sun)** section and select the box that appears below it.
Netscape 7.1 or higher	1. Select **Edit → Preferences**. 2. Select **Advanced**. 3. Select **Scripts & Plugins**. 4. Make sure the **Navigator** box is checked to **Enable JavaScript**. 5. Click **OK**.
Mozilla 1.4 or higher	1. Select **Tools**. 2. Select **Web Features**. 3. Select the boxes next to **Enable Java** and **Enable JavaScript**.

Set Cache to Always Reload a Page

Browser	Steps
Internet Explorer (IE) 6.0 or higher	1. Select **Tools → Internet Options**. 2. Select **General** tab. 3. Go to the **Temporary Internet Files** and click the **Settings** button. 4. Select the radio button for **Every visit to the page** and click **OK** when complete.
Netscape 7.1 or higher	1. Select **Edit → Preferences**. 2. Select **Advanced**. 3. Select **Cache**. 4. Select the **Every time I view the page** radio button. 5. Click **OK**.
Mozilla 1.4 or higher	1. Select **Tools**. 2. Select **Privacy**. 3. Expand the **Cache** section and designate a disk space number if one isn't in place already.

Plug-Ins

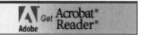 **Adobe Acrobat Reader**—With the free Acrobat Reader software you can view and print Adobe PDF files. Many Evolve products offer student and instructor manuals, checklists, and more in this format!

Download at: *http://www.adobe.com*

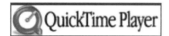 **Apple QuickTime**—Install this to hear word pronunciations, heart and lung sounds, and many other helpful audio clips within Evolve Online Courses!

Download at: *http://www.apple.com*

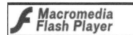 **Macromedia Flash Player**—This player will enhance your viewing of many Evolve web pages, as well as educational short-form to long-form animation within the Evolve Learning System!

Download at: *http://www.macromedia.com*

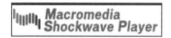 **Macromedia Shockwave Player**—Shockwave is best for viewing the many interactive learning activities within Evolve Online Courses!

Download at: *http://www.macromedia.com*

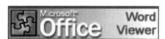 **Microsoft Word Viewer**—With this viewer Microsoft Word users can share documents with those who don't have Word, and users without Word can open and view Word documents. Many Evolve products have testbank, student and instructor manuals, and other documents available for downloading and viewing on your own computer!

Download at: *http://www.microsoft.com*

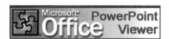 **Microsoft PowerPoint Viewer**—View PowerPoint 97, 2000, and 2002 presentations even if you don't have PowerPoint with this viewer. Many Evolve products have slides available for downloading and viewing on your own computer!

Download at: *http://www.microsoft.com*

SUPPORT INFORMATION

Live support is available to customers in the United States and Canada from 7:30 a.m. to 7:00 p.m. (Central Time), Monday through Friday by calling, **1-800-401-9962**. You can also send an email to evolve-support@elsevier.com.

There is also **24/7 support information** available on the Evolve website (http://evolve.elsevier.com), including:

- Guided Tours
- Tutorials
- Frequently Asked Questions (FAQs)
- Online Copies of Course User Guides
- And much more!

A QUICK TOUR

Welcome to *Virtual Clinical Excursions—Medical-Surgical*, a virtual hospital setting in which you can work with multiple complex patient simulations and also learn to access and evaluate the information resources that are essential for high-quality patient care.

The virtual hospital, Pacific View Regional Hospital, has realistic architecture and access to patient rooms, a Nurses' Station, and a Medication Room.

■ BEFORE YOU START

Make sure you have your textbook nearby when you use the *Virtual Clinical Excursions—Medical-Surgical* CD. You will want to consult topic areas in your textbook frequently while working with the CD and using this workbook.

■ HOW TO SIGN IN

- Enter your name on the Student Nurse identification badge.
- Now click the down arrow next to **Select Period of Care**. This drop-down menu gives you four periods of care from which to choose. In Periods of Care 1 through 3, you can actively engage in patient assessment, entry of data in the electronic patient record (EPR), and medication administration. Period of Care 4 presents the day in review. Highlight and click the appropriate period of care. (For this quick tour, choose **Period of Care 2**.)
- Click **Go** in the lower right side of the screen.
- This takes you to the Patient List screen (see example on page 11). Only the patients on the floor you choose (Medical-Surgical) are available. Note that the virtual time is provided in the box at the lower left corner of the screen (1115, since we chose Period of Care 2).

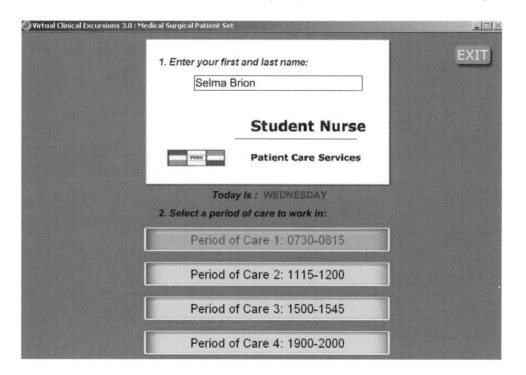

■ PATIENT LIST

MEDICAL-SURGICAL UNIT

Harry George (Room 401)
Osteomyelitis—A middle-aged Caucasian male admitted from a homeless shelter with an infected leg. He has complications of type 2 diabetes mellitus, alcohol abuse, nicotine addiction, poor pain control, and complex psychosocial issues.

Jacquline Catanazaro (Room 402)
Asthma—A middle-aged Caucasian female admitted with an acute asthma exacerbation and suspected pneumonia. She has complications of chronic schizophrenia, noncompliance with medication therapy, obesity, and herniated disc.

Piya Jordan (Room 403)
Bowel obstruction—An older Asian female admitted with a colon mass and suspected adenocarcinoma. She undergoes a right hemicolectomy. This patient's complications include atrial fibrillation, hypokalemia, and symptoms of meperidine toxicity.

Clarence Hughes (Room 404)
Degenerative joint disease—An older African-American male admitted for a left total knee replacement. His preparations for discharge are complicated by the development of a pulmonary embolus and the need for ongoing intravenous therapy.

Pablo Rodriguez (Room 405)
Metastatic lung carcinoma—An older Hispanic male admitted with symptoms of dehydration and malnutrition. He has chronic pain secondary to multiple subcutaneous skin nodules and psychosocial concerns related to family issues with his approaching death.

Patricia Newman (Room 406)
Pneumonia—A middle-aged female admitted with worsening pulmonary function and an acute respiratory infection. Her chronic emphysema is complicated by heavy smoking, hypertension, and malnutrition. She needs access to community resources such as a smoking cessation program and meal assistance.

■ HOW TO SELECT A PATIENT

- You can choose one or more patients to work with from the Patient List by clicking the box to the left of the patient name(s). (In order to receive a scorecard for a patient, the patient must be selected before proceeding to the Nurses' Station.)
- Click on **Get Report** to the right of the medical records number (MRN) to view a summary of the patient's care during the 12-hour period before your arrival on the unit.
- When you are ready to begin your care, click on **Go to Nurses' Station** in the right lower corner.

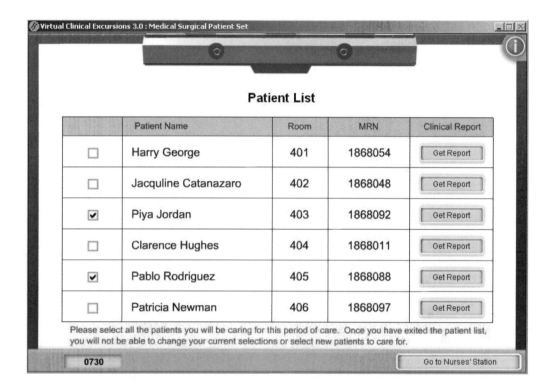

■ HOW TO FIND A PATIENT'S RECORDS

NURSES' STATION

Within the Nurses' Station, you will see:

1. A clipboard that contains the patient list for that floor.
2. A chart rack with patient charts labeled by room number, a notebook labeled Kardex, and a notebook labeled MAR (Medication Administration Record).
3. A desktop computer with access to the Electronic Patient Record (EPR).
4. A tool bar across the top of the screen that can also be used to access the Patient List, EPR, Chart, MAR, and Kardex. This tool bar is also accessible from each patient's room.
5. A Drug Guide containing information about the medications you are able to administer to your patients.

As you run your cursor over an item, it will be highlighted. To select, simply double-click on the item. As you use these resources, you will always be able to return to the Nurses' Station by clicking on the **Return to Nurses' Station** bar located in the right lower corner of your screen.

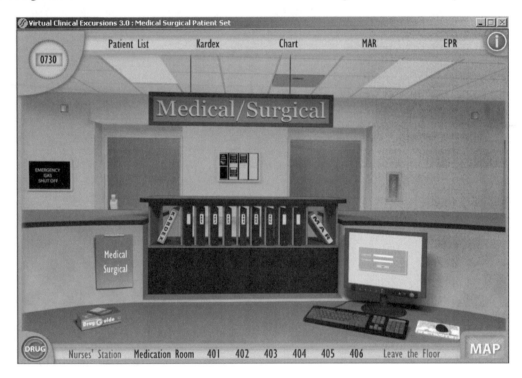

MEDICATION ADMINISTRATION RECORD (MAR)

The MAR icon located in the tool bar at the top of your screen accesses current 24-hour medications for each patient. Click on the icon and the MAR will open. (*Note:* You can also access the MAR by clicking on the blue MAR notebook on the far right side of the book rack in the center of the screen.) Within the MAR, tabs on the right side of the screen allow you to select patients by room number. Be careful to make sure you select the correct tab number for *your* patient rather than simply reading the first record that appears after the MAR opens. Each MAR sheet lists the following:

- Medications
- Route and dosage of medications
- Times of administration of medication

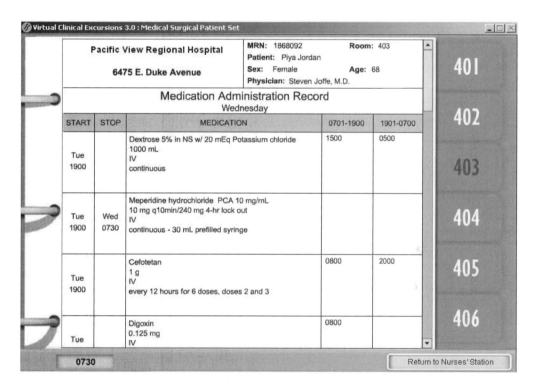

Note: The MAR changes each day. Expired MARs are stored in the patients' charts.

CHARTS

To access patient charts, either click on the **Chart** icon at the top of your screen or anywhere within the chart rack in the center of the Nurses' Station screen. When the close-up view appears, the individual charts are labeled by room number. To open a chart, click on the room number of the patient whose chart you wish to review. The patient's name and allergies will appear, along with a list of tabs on the right side of the screen, allowing you to view the following data:

- Allergies
- Physician's Orders
- Physician's Notes
- Nurse's Notes
- Laboratory Reports
- Diagnostic Reports
- Surgical Reports
- Consultations

- Patient Education
- History and Physical
- Nursing Admission
- Expired MARs
- Consents
- Mental Health
- Admissions
- Emergency Department

Information appears in real time. The entries are in reverse chronological order, so use the down arrow at the right side of the chart page to scroll down to view previous entries. Flip from tab to tab to view multiple data fields or click on the **Return to Nurses' Station** bar in the lower right corner of the screen to exit the chart.

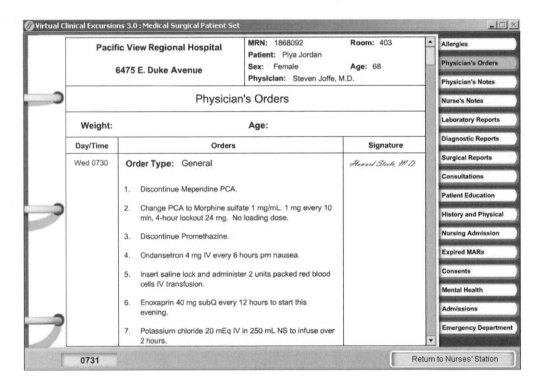

ELECTRONIC PATIENT RECORD (EPR)

The EPR can be accessed from the computer in the Nurses' Station or from the EPR icon located in the tool bar at the top of your screen. To access a patient's EPR:

- Click on either the computer screen or the **EPR** icon.
- Your user name and password are automatically filled in.
- Click on **Login** to enter the EPR.

The EPR used in Pacific View Regional Hospital represents a composite of commercial versions being used in hospitals. You can access the EPR:

- for a patient (by room number).
- to review existing data.
- to enter data you collect while working with a patient.

The EPR is updated daily, so no matter what day or part of a shift you are working, there will be a current EPR with the patient's data from the past days of the current hospital stay. This type of simulated EPR allows you to examine how data for different attributes have changed over time, as well as to examine data for all of a patient's attributes at a particular time. The EPR is fully functional (as it is in a real-life hospital). You can enter such data as blood pressure, breath sounds, and certain treatments. The EPR will not, however, allow you to enter data for a previous time period. Use the arrows at the bottom of the screen to move forward and backward in time.

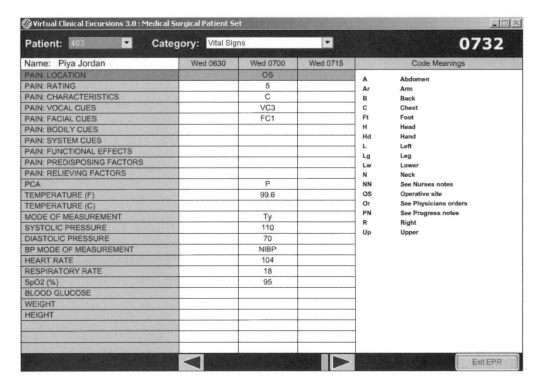

Name: Piya Jordan	Wed 0630	Wed 0700	Wed 0715	Code Meanings	
PAIN: LOCATION		OS		A	Abdomen
PAIN: RATING		5		Ar	Arm
PAIN: CHARACTERISTICS		C		B	Back
PAIN: VOCAL CUES		VC3		C	Chest
PAIN: FACIAL CUES		FC1		Ft	Foot
PAIN: BODILY CUES				H	Head
PAIN: SYSTEM CUES				Hd	Hand
PAIN: FUNCTIONAL EFFECTS				L	Left
PAIN: PREDISPOSING FACTORS				Lg	Leg
PAIN: RELIEVING FACTORS				Lw	Lower
PCA		P		N	Neck
TEMPERATURE (F)		99.6		NN	See Nurses notes
TEMPERATURE (C)				OS	Operative site
MODE OF MEASUREMENT		Ty		Or	See Physicians orders
SYSTOLIC PRESSURE		110		PN	See Progress notes
DIASTOLIC PRESSURE		70		R	Right
BP MODE OF MEASUREMENT		NIBP		Up	Upper
HEART RATE		104			
RESPIRATORY RATE		18			
SpO2 (%)		95			
BLOOD GLUCOSE					
WEIGHT					
HEIGHT					

At the top of the EPR screen, you can choose patients by their room numbers. In addition, you have access to 17 different categories of patient data. To change patients or data categories, click the down arrow to the right of the room number or category.

The categories of patient data in the EPR as as follows:

- Vital Signs
- Respiratory
- Cardiovascular
- Neurologic
- Gastrointestinal
- Excretory
- Musculoskeletal
- Integumentary
- Reproductive
- Psychosocial
- Wounds and Drains
- Activity
- Hygiene and Comfort
- Safety
- Nutrition
- IV
- Intake and Output

Remember, each hospital selects its own codes. The codes used in the EPR at Pacific View Regional Hospital may be different from ones you have seen in clinical rotations that have computerized patient records. Take some time to acquaint yourself with the codes. Within the Vital Signs category, click on any item in the left column (e.g., heart rate). In the far-right column, you will see a list of code meanings for the possible findings and/or descriptors for that assessment area.

You will use the codes to record the data you collect as you work with patients. Click on the box in the last time column to the right of the data and wait for the code meanings applicable to that entry to appear. Select the appropriate code to describe your assessment findings and type it in the box. (*Note:* If no cursor appears within the box, click on the box again until the blue shading disappears and the blinking cursor appears.) Once the data are typed in this box, they are entered into the patient's record for this period of care only.

To leave the EPR, click on **Exit EPR** in the bottom right corner of the screen.

■ **VISITING A PATIENT**

From the Nurses' Station, click on the room number of the patient you wish to visit in the tool bar at the bottom of your screen. Once you are inside the room, you will see a still photo of your patient in the top left corner. To verify that this is the patient you have chosen, click on the **Check Armband** icon to the right of the photo. The patient's identification data will appear. If you click on **Check Allergies** (the next icon to the right), a list of the patient's allergies (if any) will replace the photo.

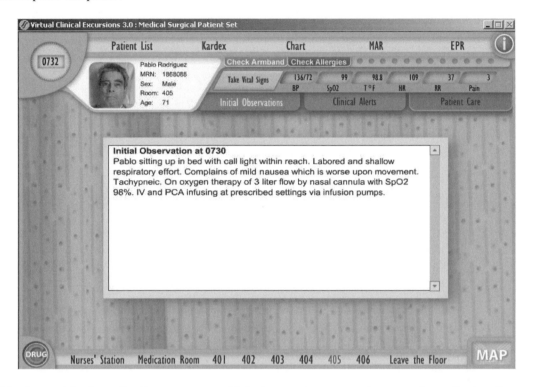

Also located in the patient's room are multiple icons you may use to assess the patient or the patient's medications. A clock is provided in the upper left corner of the room to monitor your progress in real time.

• The tool bar across the top of the screen allows you to check the **Patient List**, access the **EPR** to check or enter data, and view the patient's **Chart**, **MAR**, or **Kardex**.

• The **Take Vital Signs** icon allows you to measure the patient's up-to-the-minute blood pressure, oxygen saturation, temperature, heart rate, respiratory rate, and pain level.

• When you click on **Initial Observations**, a description appears in the text box under the patient's photo, allowing you a "look" at the patient as if you had just stepped in. To the right of this icon is **Clinical Alerts**, a resource that allows you to make decisions about priority medication interventions based on emerging data collected in real time. Check this screen throughout your period of care to avoid missing critical information related to recently ordered or STAT medications.

• Clicking on the **Patient Care** icon opens up three specific learning environments within the patient room: **Physical Assessment**, **Nurse-Client Interactions**, and **Medication Administration**.

• To perform a **Physical Assessment**, choose a body area (such as **Head & Neck**) by clicking on the appropriate icon in the column of yellow buttons. This activates a list of system subcategories for that body area (e.g., see **Sensory**, **Neurologic**, etc. in the green boxes). After you click on the system that you wish to evaluate, a still photo and text box appear, describing the assessment findings. The still photo is a "snapshot" of how an assessment of this area might be done or what the finding might look like. For every body area, there is also an **Equipment** button located on the far right of the screen.

- To the right of the Physical Assessment icon is **Nurse-Client Interactions**. Clicking on this icon will reveal the times and titles of any videos available for viewing. (*Note:* If the video you wish to see is not listed, this means you have not yet reached the correct virtual time to view that video. Check the virtual clock; you may return to access the video once its designated time has occurred—as long as you do so within the corresponding period of care.) To view a listed video, click on the white arrow to the right of the video title. Use the square control buttons below the video to start, stop, pause, rewind, or fast-forward the action or to mute the sound.

- **Medication Administration** is the pathway that allows you to review and administer medications to a patient after you have prepared them in the Medication Room. This process is addressed further in the *How to Prepare Medications* section (pages 19-20) and in *Medications* (pages 26-30). For additional hands-on practice, see *Reducing Medication Errors* (pages 37-41).

■ HOW TO QUIT, CHANGE PATIENTS, OR CHANGE PERIOD OF CARE

How to Quit: From most screens, you may click the **Leave the Floor** icon on the bottom tool bar to the right of the patient room numbers. (*Note:* From some screens, you will first need to click an **Exit** button or **Return to Nurses' Station** before clicking **Leave the Floor**.) When the Floor Menu appears, click **Exit** to leave the program.

How to Change Patients or Period of Care: To change patients, simply click on the new patient's room number. (You cannot receive a scorecard for a new patient, however, unless you have already selected that patient on the Patient List screen.) To change to a new period of care or restart the virtual clock for a new patient, click the **Leave the Floor** icon and then **Restart**.

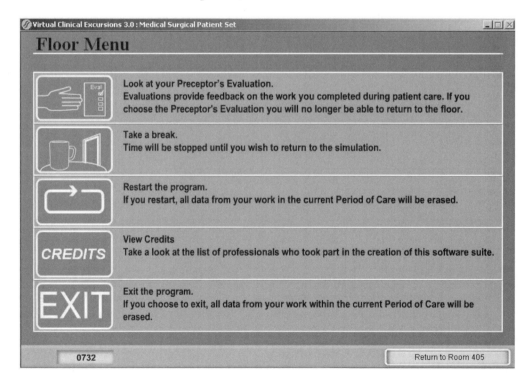

■ HOW TO PREPARE MEDICATIONS

From the Nurses' Station or the patient's room, you can access the Medication Room by clicking on the icon in the tool bar at the bottom of your screen to the left of the patient room numbers.

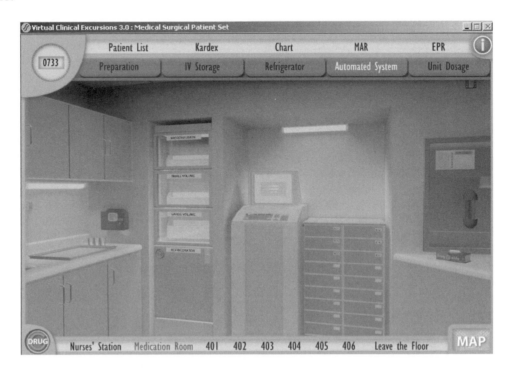

In the Medication Room you have access to the following (from left to right):

- A preparation area is located on the counter under the cabinets. To begin the medication preparation process, click on the tray on the counter or click on the **Preparation** icon at the top of the screen. The next screen leads you through a preparation sequence (called the Preparation Wizard) to prepare medications one at a time for administration to a patient. However, no medication has been selected at this time. We will do this while working with a patient in *A Detailed Tour*. To exit this screen, click on **View the Medication Room**.

- To the right of the cabinets (and above the refrigerator), IV storage bins are provided. Click on the bins themselves or on the **IV Storage** icon at the top of the screen. The bins are labeled **Microinfusion**, **Small Volume**, and **Large Volume**. Click on an individual bin to see a list of its contents. No medications are available in the bins at this time, but if they were, you could click on an individual medication and its label would appear to the right under the patient's name. Next, you would click **Put Medication on Tray**. If you ever change your mind or choose the incorrect medication, you can reverse your actions by clicking on **Put Medication in Bin**. Click **Close Bin** in the right bottom corner to exit. **View Medication Room** brings you back to a full view of the entire room.

- A refrigerator is located under the IV storage bins to hold any medications that must be stored below room temperature. Click on it to remove your medications; then click **Close Door**. You can also access this area by clicking the **Refrigerator** icon at the top of the screen.

- To prepare controlled substances, click the **Automated System** icon at the top of the screen or click the computer monitor located to the right of the IV storage bins. A login screen will appear; your name and password are automatically filled in. Click **Login**. Select a patient to log medications out for; then select the drawer you wish to open. Click **Open Drawer**, choose **Put Medication on Tray**, and then click **Close Drawer**.

- Next to the Automated System is a set of drawers identified by patient room number. To access these, click on the drawers themselves or on the **Unit Dosage** icon at the top of the screen. This provides a close-up view of the drawers. Click on the room number of the patient you are working with to open that drawer. Next, click on the medication you would like to prepare for the patient, and a label appears to the right under the patient's name, listing strength, units, and dosage per unit. You can **Open** and **Close** this medication label by clicking the appropriate icon. To exit, click **Close Drawer**; then click **View Medication Room**.

At any time, you can learn about a medication you wish to prepare for a patient by clicking on the **Drug** icon in the bottom left corner of the medication room screen or by clicking the **Drug Guide** book on the counter to the right of the unit dosage drawers. The **Drug Guide** provides information about the medications commonly included in nursing drug handbooks. Nutritional supplements and maintenance intravenous fluid preparations are not included.

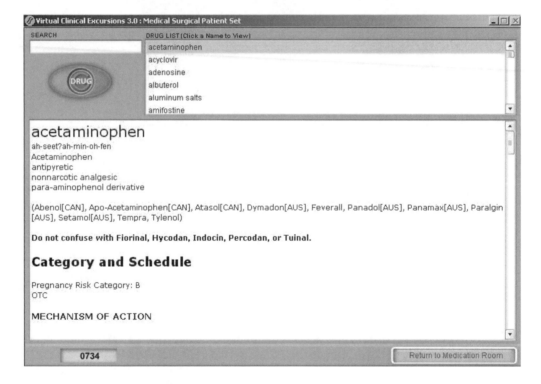

To access the MAR to review the medications ordered for a patient, click on the **MAR** icon located in the tool bar at the top of your screen. You may also click the **Review MAR** icon in the tool bar at the bottom of your screen from inside each medication storage area.

After you have chosen and prepared your medications, return to the patient's room to administer them by clicking on the room number in the bottom tool bar. Once inside the patient's room, click on **Medication Administration** and follow the administration sequence.

■ PRECEPTOR'S EVALUATIONS

When you have finished a session, click on **Leave the Floor** to go to the Floor Menu. At this point, you can click on the icon next to **Look at your Preceptor's Evaluation** to receive a scorecard that provides feedback on the work you completed during patient care.

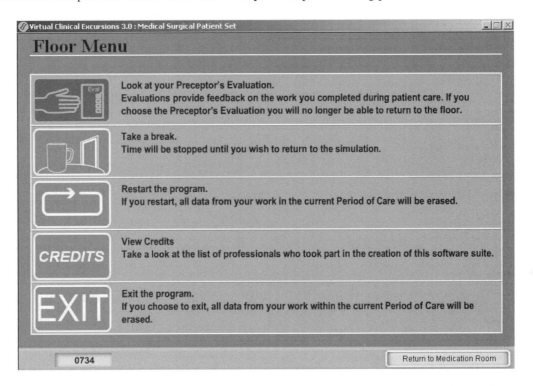

Evaluations are available for each patient you signed in for. Click on any of the **Medication Scorecard** icons to see an example. The scorecard compares the medications you administered to a patient during a period of care with what should have been administered. Table A lists the correct medications. Table B lists any medications that were administered incorrectly.

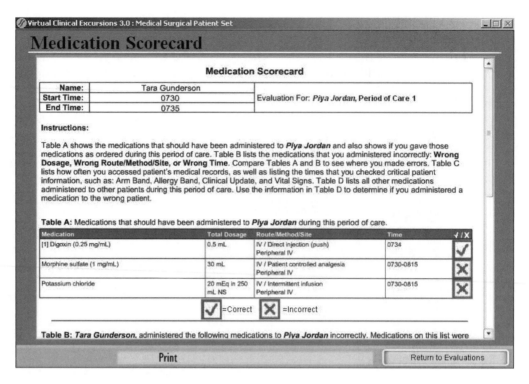

Not every medication listed on the MAR should be given. For example, a patient might have an allergy to a drug that was ordered, or a medication might have been improperly transcribed to the MAR. Predetermined medication "errors" embedded within the program challenge you to exercise critical thinking skills and professional judgment when deciding to administer a medication, just as you would in a real hospital. Use all your available resources, such as the patient's chart and the MAR, to make your decision.

Table C lists the resources that were available to assist you in medication administration, and it documents whether and when you accessed these resources. For example, did you check the patient armband or perform a check of vital signs? If so, when?

You can click **Print** to get a copy of this report if needed. Click **Return to Evaluations** when finished.

■ FLOOR MAP

To get a general sense of your location within the hospital, click on the **Map** icon found in the lower right corner of most of the screens in the *Virtual Clinical Excursions—Medical-Surgical* program. A floor map will appear, showing the layout of the floor you are currently on, as well as a directory of the patients and services on that floor. As you move your cursor over the directory list, the location of each room is highlighted (and vice versa). The floor map can be accessed from the Nurses' Station, Medication Room, and each patient's room.

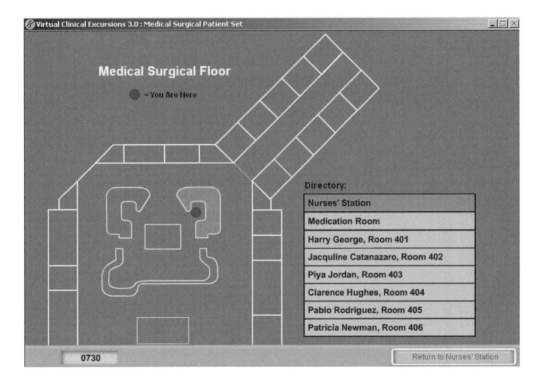

A DETAILED TOUR

If you wish to more thoroughly understand the capabilities of *Virtual Clinical Excursions—Medical-Surgical*, take a detailed tour by completing the following section. During this tour, we will work with a specific patient to introduce you to all the different components and learning opportunities available within the software.

■ WORKING WITH A PATIENT

Sign in and select the Medical-Surgical floor for Period of Care 1 (0730-0815). From the Patient List, select Piya Jordan in Room 403; however, do not go to the Nurses' Station yet.

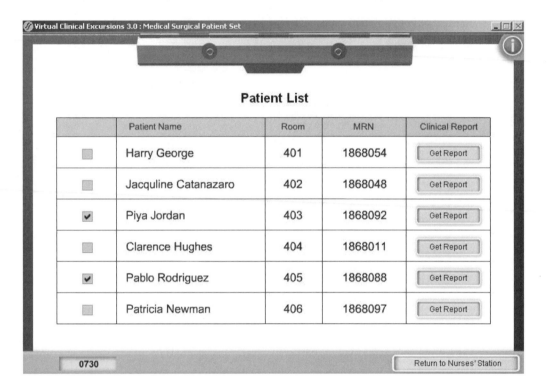

■ REPORT

In hospitals, when one shift ends and another begins, the outgoing nurse who attended a patient will give a verbal and sometimes a written summary of that patient's condition to the incoming nurse who will assume care for the patient. This summary is called a report and is an important source of data to provide an overview of a patient. Your first task is to get clinical report on Piya Jordan. To do this, click **Get Report** in the far right column in this patient's row. From this summary, identify the problems and areas of concern that you will need to address for this patient.

When you have finished reading the report and noting any areas of concern, click **Go to Nurses' Station**.

■ CHARTS

You can access Piya Jordan's chart from the Nurses' Station or from the patient's room (403). We will access it from the Nurses' Station: Click on the chart rack or on the **Chart** icon in the tool bar at the top of your screen. Next, click on the chart labeled **403** to open the medical record for Piya Jordan. Click on the **Emergency Department** tab to view a record of why this patient was admitted.

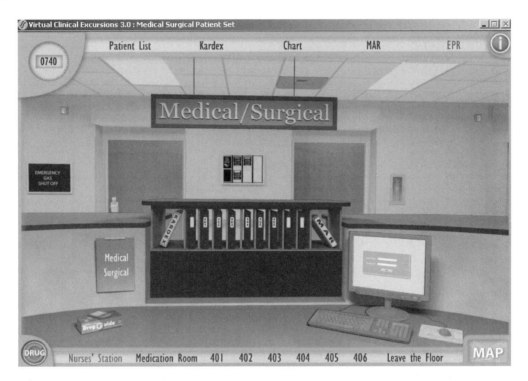

How many days has Piya Jordan been in the hospital?

What tests were done upon her arrival in the Emergency Department and why?

What was her reason for admission?

You should also click on **Surgical Reports** to learn what procedures were performed and when. Finally, review the **Nursing Admission** and **History and Physical** tabs to view information on the health history of this patient. When you are done reviewing the chart, click **Return to Nurses' Station**.

■ MEDICATIONS

Open the Medication Administration Record (MAR) by clicking on the **MAR** icon in the tool bar at the top of your screen. *Remember:* The MAR automatically opens to the first occupied room number on the floor (in this case, Room 401, Harry George). Since you need to access Piya Jordan's MAR, click on tab **403** (her room number). Always make sure you are giving the *Right Drug to the Right Patient!*

Examine the list of medications prescribed for Piya Jordan. Write down the medications that need to be given during this period of care (0730-0815). For each medication, note the dosage, route, and time in the chart below.

Time	Medication	Dosage	Route
0800	Digoxin	0.125 mg	IV

Click on **Return to Nurses' Station**. Next, click on **403** on the bottom tool bar and then verify that you are indeed in Piya Jordan's room. Select **Clinical Alerts** (the icon to the right of Initial Observations) to check for any emerging data that might affect your medication administration priorities. Go to the patient's chart (click on the **Chart** icon; then click on **403**). When the chart opens, select the **Physician's Orders** tab.

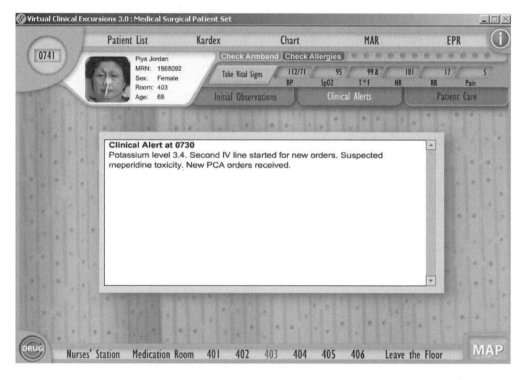

Review the orders. Have any new medications been ordered? Return to the MAR (click **Return to Room 403**; then click **MAR**). Verify that the new medications have been correctly transcribed to the MAR. Mistakes are sometimes made in the transcription process in the hospital setting, and it is sound practice to double-check any new order.

Are there any patient assessments you will need to perform before administering these medications? If so, return to Room 403 and click on **Review of Systems** to complete those before proceeding. (*Hint:* Check apical pulse.)

Now click on the **Medication Room** icon in the tool bar at the bottom of your screen to locate and prepare the medications for Piya Jordan.

In the Medication Room, you must access the medications for Piya Jordan from the specific dispensing system in which each medication is stored. Locate each medication that needs to be given in this time period and click on **Put Medication on Tray** as appropriate. (*Hint:* Look in Unit Dosage drawer first.) When you are finished, click on **Close Drawer** and then on **View Medication Room**. Now click on the medication tray on the counter on the left side of the medication room screen to begin preparing the medications you have selected. (*Note:* Instead of clicking on the tray, you can click **Preparation** at top of screen.)

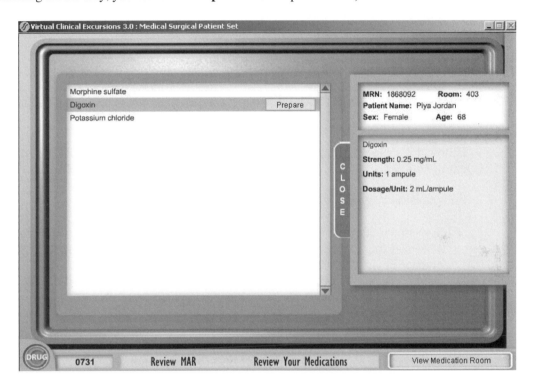

In the preparation area, you should see a list of the medications you put on the tray in the previous steps. Click on the first medication and then click **Prepare**. Follow the onscreen instructions of the Preparation Wizard, providing any data requested. As an example, let's follow the preparation process for digoxin, one of the medications due to be administered to Piya Jordan during this period of care. To begin, click to select **Digoxin**; then click **Prepare**. Now work through the Preparation Wizard sequence as detailed below:

> Amount of medication in the ampule: 2 mL
> Enter the amount of medication you will draw up into a syringe: **0.5** mL
> Click **Next**.
> Select the patient you wish to set aside the medication for:
> Click **Room 403, Piya Jordan**.
> Click **Finish**.
> Click **Return to Medication Room**.

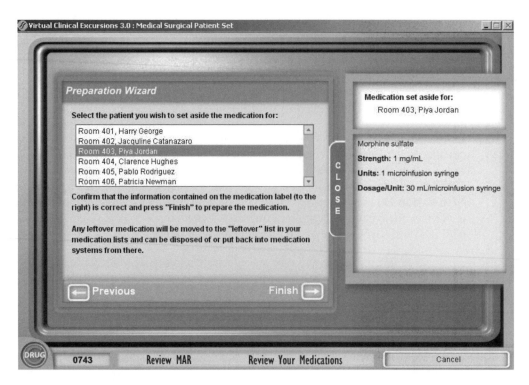

Follow this same basic process for the other medications due to be administered to Piya Jordan during this period of care. (*Hint:* Look in **IV Storage** and **Automated System**.)

PREPARATION WIZARD EXCEPTIONS

- Some medications in *Virtual Clinical Excursions—Medical-Surgical* are prepepared by the pharmacy (e.g., IV antibiotics) and taken to the patient room as a whole. This is common practice in most hospitals.
- Blood products are not administered by students through the *Virtual Clinical Excursions—Medical-Surgical* simulations since blood administration follows specific protocols not covered in this program.
- The *Virtual Clinical Excursions—Medical-Surgical* simulations do not allow for mixing more than one type of medication, such as regular and Lente insulins, in the same syringe. In the clinical setting, when multiple types of insulin are ordered for a patient, the regular insulin is drawn up first, followed by the longer-acting insulin. Insulin is always administered in a special unit-marked syringe.

Now return to Room 403 (click on **403** on bottom tool bar) to administer Piya Jordan's medications.

At any time during the medication administration process, you can perform a further review of systems, take vital signs, check information contained within the chart, or verify patient identity and allergies. Inside Piya Jordan's room, click **Take Vital Signs**. (*Note:* These findings change over time to reflect the temporal changes you would find in a patient similar to Piya Jordan.)

When you have gathered all the data you need, click on **Patient Care** and then select **Medication Administration**. After reviewing your medications, continue the administration process with the digoxin ordered for Piya Jordan. In the list of medications set aside for this patient, click to highlight **Digoxin**. Next, click on the down arrow to the right of **Select** and choose **Administer** from the drop-down menu. This will activate the Administration Wizard. Complete the Wizard sequence as follows:

- Route: **IV**
- Method: **Direct Injection**
- Site: **Peripheral IV**
- Click **Administer to Patient** arrow.
- Would you like to document this administration in the MAR? **Yes**
- Click **Finish** arrow.

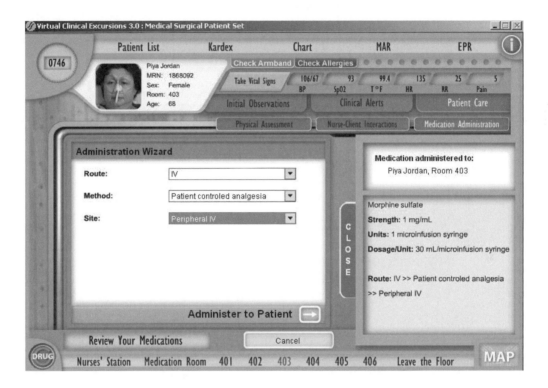

Selections are recorded by a tracking system and evaluated on a Medication Scorecard stored under Preceptor's Evaluations. This scorecard can be viewed, printed, and given to your instructor. To access the Preceptor's Evaluations, click on **Leave the Floor**. When the Floor Menu appears, click on the icon next to **Look at Your Preceptor's Evaluation**. From the list of evaluations, click on **Medication Scorecard** inside the box with Piya Jordan's name.

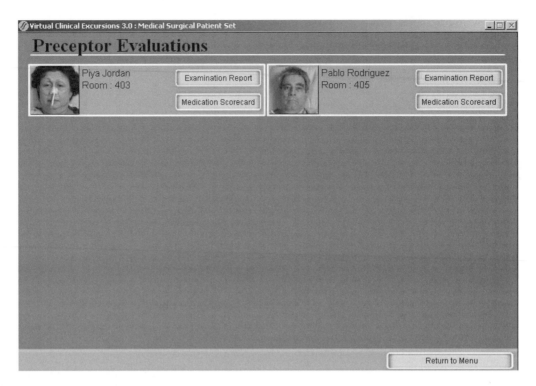

■ MEDICATION SCORECARD

- First, review Table A. Was digoxin given correctly? Did you give the other medications as ordered?
- Table B shows you which (if any) medications you gave incorrectly.
- Table C addresses the resources used for Piya Jordan. Did you access the patient's chart, MAR, EPR, or Kardex as needed to make safe medication administration decisions?
- Did you check the patient's armband to verify her identity? Did you check whether your patient had any known allergies to medications? Were vital signs taken?

Now that you understand the basic steps of medication preparation and administration, the following section will allow you to practice these skills further—with an increased emphasis on reducing medication errors by using the Medication Scorecard to evaluate your work.

■ VITAL SIGNS

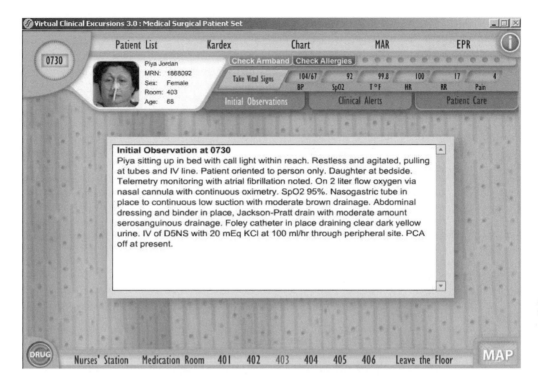

Vital signs, often considered the traditional signs of life, include body temperature, heart rate, respiratory rate, blood pressure, oxygen saturation of the blood, and the patient's experience of pain.

Inside Piya Jordan's room, click **Take Vital Signs**. (*Remember:* You can take vital signs at any time. The data change over time to reflect the temporal changes you would find in a patient similar to Piya Jordan.) Collect vital signs for this patient and record them in the following table. Note the time at which you collected each of these data.

Vital Signs	Findings/Time
Blood pressure	
O$_2$ saturation	
Heart rate	
Respiratory rate	
Temperature	
Pain rating	

After you are done, click on the **EPR** icon located in the tool bar at the top of the screen.

Complete the EPR Login screen as directed in *A Quick Tour* (see page 15 of this workbook). Click on the down arrow next to Patient and choose Piya Jordan's room number **403**. Select **Vital Signs** as the category. Next, record the vital signs data you just collected in the last column. (*Note:* If you need help with this process, see page 16.) Now compare these findings with the data you collected earlier for this patient's vital signs. Use these earlier findings to establish a baseline for each of the vital signs.

  a. Are any of the data you collected significantly different from the baseline for a particular vital sign?

      Circle One: Yes   No

  b. If "Yes," which data are different?

■ PHYSICAL ASSESSMENT

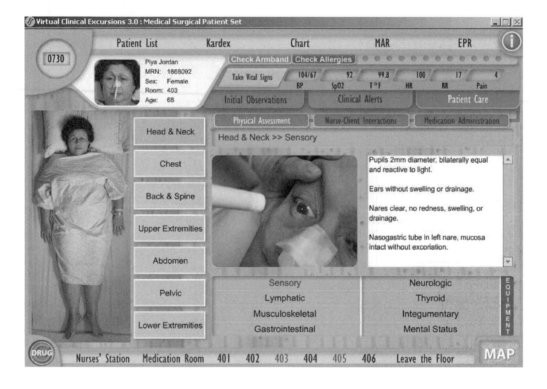

After you have finished examining the EPR for vital signs, click **Exit EPR** to return to Room 403. Click **Patient Care** and then **Physical Assessment**. Think about what information you received in report, as well as what you may have learned about this patient from the chart. What area(s) of examination should you pay most attention to at this time? Is there any equipment you should be monitoring? Conduct a physical assessment of the body areas and systems that you consider priorities for Piya Jordan. For example, select **Head & Neck**; then click on and assess **Sensory** and **Lymphatic**. Complete any other assessment(s) you think are necessary at this time. In the following table, record the data you collected during this examination.

Area of Examination	Findings
Head & Neck Sensory	
Head & Neck Lymphatic	

After you have finished collecting these data, return to the EPR. Compare the data that were already in the record with those you just collected.

    a.   Are any of the data you collected significantly different from the baselines for this patient?

        Circle One: Yes   No

    b.   If "Yes," which data are different?

■ **NURSE-CLIENT INTERACTIONS**

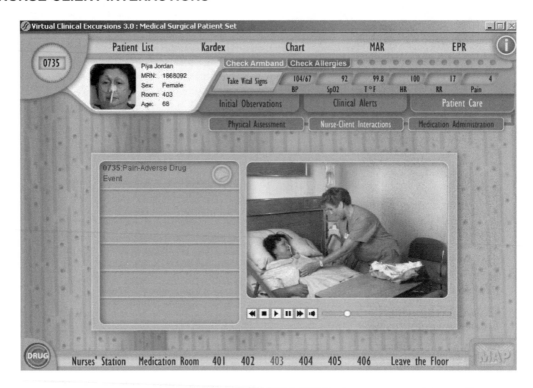

Click on **Patient Care** from inside Piya Jordan's room (403). Now click on **Nurse-Client Interactions** to access a short video titled **Pain—Adverse Drug Event**, which is available for viewing at 0735 (based on the virtual clock in the upper left corner of your screen). To begin the video, click on the arrow next to its title. You will observe a nurse communicating with Piya Jordan and her daughter. There are many variations of nursing practice, some exemplifying "best" practice and some not. Note whether the nurse in this interaction displays professional behavior and compassionate care. Are her words congruent with what is going on with the patient? Does this interaction "feel right" to you? If not, how would you handle this situation differently? Explain.

Note: If the video you wish to view is not listed, this means you have not yet reached the correct virtual time to view that video. Check the virtual clock; you may return to access the video once its designated time has occurred—as long as you do so within the corresponding period of care.

At least one Nurse-Client Interactions video is available during each period of care. Viewing these videos can help you learn more about what is occurring with a patient at a certain time and also prompt you to discriminate between nurse communications that are ideal and those that need improvement. Compassionate care and the ability to communicate clearly are essential components of delivering quality nursing care, and it is during your clinical time that you will begin to refine these skills.

■ COLLECTING AND EVALUATING DATA

Each of the activities you perform in the Patient Care environment generates a great deal of assessment data. Remember that after you collect data, you can record your findings in the EPR. You can also review the EPR, patient's chart, videos, and MAR at any time. You will get plenty of practice collecting and then evaluating data in context of the patient's course.

Now, here's an important question for you:

> Did the previous sequence of exercises provide the most efficient way to assess Piya Jordan?

For example, you went to the patient's room to get vital signs, then back to the EPR to enter data and compare your findings with extant data. Next, you went back to the patient's room to do a physical examination, then again back to the EPR to enter and review data. If this back-and-forth process of data collection and recording seemed inefficient, remember the following:

- Plan all of your nursing activities to maximize efficiency while at the same time optimizing quality of patient care. (Think about what data you might need to perform certain tasks. For example, do you need to check a heart rate before administering a cardiac medication or check an IV site before starting an infusion?)

- You collect a tremendous amount of data when you work with a patient. Very few people can accurately remember all these data for more than a few minutes. Develop efficient assessment skills, and record data as soon as possible after collecting them.

- Assessment data are only the starting point for the nursing process.

Make a clear distinction between these first exercises and how you actually provide nursing care. These initial exercises were designed to involve you actively in the use of different software components. This workbook focuses on sensible practices for implementing the nursing process in ways that ensure the highest quality care of patients.

Most important, remember that a human being changes through time, and that these changes include both the physical and psychosocial facets of a person as a living organism. Think about this for a moment. Some patients may change physically in a very short time (a patient with emerging myocardial infarction) or more slowly (a patient with a chronic illness). Patients' overall physical and psychosocial conditions may improve or deteriorate. They may have effective coping skills and familial support, or they may feel alone and full of despair. In fact, each individual is a complex mix of physical and psychosocial elements, and at least some of these elements usually change through time.

Thus it is crucial *not* to think of the nursing process as a simple one-time, five-step procedure:

- Assessment
- Nursing Diagnosis
- Planning
- Implementation
- Evaluation

Rather, the nursing process should be utilized as a creative and systematic approach to delivering nursing care. Furthermore, because all living organisms are constantly changing, we must apply the nursing process over and over. Each time we follow the nursing process for an individual patient, we refine our understanding of that patient's physical and psychosocial conditions based on collection and analysis of many different types of data. *Virtual Clinical Excursions—Medical-Surgical* will help you develop both the creativity and the systematic approach needed to become a nurse who is equipped to deliver the highest quality care to all patients.

REDUCING MEDICATION ERRORS

Earlier in this detailed tour, you learned the basic steps of medication preparation and administration. The following simulations will allow you to practice those skills further—with an increased emphasis on reducing medication errors by using the Medication Scorecard to evaluate your work.

Sign in to work at Pacific View Regional Hospital for Period of Care 1. (*Note:* If you are already working with another patient or during another period of care, click on **Leave the Floor** and then **Restart the Program**; then sign in.)

From the Patient List, select Clarence Hughes. Then click on **Go To Nurses' Station**. Complete the following steps to prepare and administer medications to Clarence Hughes.

- Click on **Medication Room**.
- Click on **MAR** to determine prn medications that have been ordered for Clarence Hughes to address his constipation and pain. (*Note:* You may click on **Review MAR** at any time to verify correct medication order. Remember to look at the patient name on the MAR to make sure you have the correct patient's record—you must click on the correct room number within the MAR.) Click on **Return to Medication Room** after reviewing the correct MAR.
- Click on **Unit Dosage** (or on the Unit Dosage cabinet); from the close-up view, click on drawer **404**.
- Select the medications you would like to administer. After each selection, click **Put Medication on Tray**. When you are finished selecting medications, click **Close Drawer**.
- Click on **View Medication Room**.
- Click on **Automated System** (or on the Automated System unit itself). Click **Login**.
- On the next screen, specify the correct patient and drawer location.
- Select the medication you would like to administer and click on **Put Medication on Tray**. Repeat this process if you wish to administer other medications from the Automated System.
- When you are finished, click **Close Drawer**. At the bottom right corner of the next screen, click on **View Medication Room**.
- From the Medication Room, click on **Preparation** (or on the preparation tray).
- From the list of medications on your tray, choose the correct medication to administer.
- Click **Next**, specify the correct patient to administer this medication to, and click **Finish**.
- Repeat the previous two steps until all medications that you want to administer are prepared.
- You can click on **Review Your Medications** and then on **Return to Medication Room** when ready. Once you are back in the Medication Room, go directly to Clarence Hughes' room by clicking on **404** at bottom of screen.
- Inside the patient's room, administer the medication, utilizing the five rights of medication administration. After you have collected the appropriate assessment data and are ready for administration, click **Patient Care** and then **Medication Administration**. Verify that the correct patient and medication(s) appear in the left-hand window. Then click the down arrow next to Select. From the drop-down menu, select **Administer** and complete the Administration Wizard by providing any information requested. When the Wizard stops asking for information, click **Administer to Patient**. Specify **Yes** when asked whether this administration should be recorded in the MAR. Finally, click **Finish**.

■ **SELF-EVALUATION**

Now let's see how you did during your earlier medication administration!

- Click on **Leave the Floor** at the bottom of your screen. From the Floor Menu, select **Look at Your Preceptor's Evaluation**. Then click on **Medication Scorecard**.

These resources will help you find out more about each patient's medications and possible sources of medication errors.

1. Start by examining Table A. These are the medications you should have given to Clarence Hughes during this period of care. If each of the medications in Table A has a √ by it, then you made no errors. Congratulations!

If there are some medications that have an X by them, then you made one or more medication errors.

Compare Tables A and B to determine which of the following types of errors you made: Wrong Dose, Wrong Route/Method/Site, or Wrong Time. Follow these steps:
   a. Find medications in Table A that were given incorrectly.
   b. Now see if those same medications are in Table B, which shows what you actually administered to Clarence Hughes.
   c. Comparing Tables A and B, match the Strength, Dose, Route/Method/Site, and Time for each medication you administered incorrectly.
   d. Then, using the form below, list the medications given incorrectly and mark the errors you made for each medication.

Medication	Strength	Dosage	Route	Method	Site	Time
	❑	❑	❑	❑	❑	❑
	❑	❑	❑	❑	❑	❑
	❑	❑	❑	❑	❑	❑
	❑	❑	❑	❑	❑	❑

2. To help you reduce future medication errors, consider the following list of possible reasons for errors.

   - Did not check drug against MAR for correct patient, correct date, correct time, correct drug, and correct dose.
   - Did not check drug dose against MAR three times.
   - Did not open the unit dose package in the patient's room.
   - Did not correctly identify the patient using two identifiers.
   - Did not administer the drug on time.
   - Did not verify patient allergies.
   - Did not check the patient's current condition or vital sign parameters.
   - Did not consider why the patient would be receiving this drug.
   - Did not question why the drug was in the patient's drawer.
   - Did not check the physician's order and/or check with the pharmacist when there was a question about the drug or dose.
   - Did not verify that no adverse effects had occurred from a previous dose.

Based on these possibilities, determine how you made each error and record the reason into the form below:

Medication	Reason for Error

3. Look again at Table B. Are there medications listed that are not in Table A? If so, you gave a medication to Clarence Hughes that he should not have received. Complete the following exercises to help you understand how such an error might have been made.

   a. Perhaps you gave a medication that was on Clarence Hughes' MAR for this period of care, without recognizing that a change had occurred in the patient's condition that should have caused you to reconsider. Review patient records as necessary and complete the following form:

Medication	Possible Reasons Not to Give This Medication

   b. Another possibility is that you gave Clarence Hughes a medication that should have been given at a different time. Check his MAR and complete the form below to determine whether you made a Wrong Time error:

Medication	Given to Clarence Hughes at What Time	Should Have Been Given at What Time

c. Maybe you gave another patient's medication to Clarence Hughes. In this case, you made a Wrong Patient error. Check the MARs of other patients and use the form below to determine whether you made this type of error:

Medication	Given to Clarence Hughes	Should Have Been Given to

4. The Medication Scorecard provides some other interesting sources of information. For example, if there is a medication selected for Clarence Hughes but it was not given to him, there will be an X by that medication in Table A, but it will not appear in Table B. In that case, you might have given this medication to some other patient, which is another type of Wrong Patient error. To investigate further, look at Table D, which lists the medications you gave to other patients. See whether you can find any medications for Clarence Hughes that were given to another patient by mistake. Before making any decisions, be sure to cross-check the other patients' MAR because they may have had the same medication ordered. Use the following form to record your findings:

Medication	Should Have Been Given to Clarence Hughes	Given by Mistake to

REDUCING MEDICATION ERRORS 41

5. Now take some time to review the exercises you just completed. Use the form below to create an overall analysis of what you have learned. Once again, record each of the medication errors you made, including the type of each error. Then, for each error you made, indicate specifically what you would do differently to prevent this type of error from occurring again.

Medication	Type of Error	Error Prevention Tactic

Submit this form to your instructor if required as a graded assignment, or simply use these exercises to improve your understanding of medication errors and how to reduce them.

Name: _____   Date: _____

The following icons are used throughout the workbook to help you quickly identify particular activities and assignments:

 Indicates a reading assignment—tells you which textbook chapter(s) you should read before starting each lesson

 Indicates a writing activity

 Marks the beginning of an interactive CD-ROM activity—signals you to open or return to your *Virtual Clinical Excursions—Medical-Surgical* CD-ROM

 Indicates additional CD-ROM instructions

 Indicates questions and activities that require you to consult your textbook

 Indicates the approximate time required to complete an exercise

LESSON **1**

Assessment of the Patient with Osteomyelitis

👓 **Reading Assignment:** Care of the Patient with a Musculoskeletal Disorder (Chapter 4)

Patient: Harry George, Room 401

Objectives:

1. Understand the basic functions of the musculoskeletal system.
2. Review the various types of arthritis.
3. Review risk factors for osteomyelitis.
4. Identify the clinical manifestations.
5. Discuss treatment options for the patient with osteomyelitis.

Exercise 1

Writing Activity

   15 minutes

1. The skeletal system serves five major functions:

   a. The skeleton provides the body _____ that supports internal tissues and organs.

   b. The skeleton forms a _____ that protects many internal organs.

   c. Bones provide _____ for movement.

   d. The bones serve as storage areas for various _____.

   e. _____ (blood cell formation) takes place in the red bone marrow.

2. Match each type of body movement with its correct definition. (*Hint:* See Box 4-2 in your textbook.)

Type of Body Movement	Definition
_____ Abduction	a. Movement of the bone around its longitudinal axis.
_____ Adduction	b. Movement that causes the bottom of the foot to be be directed downward.
_____ Dorsiflexion	
_____ Extension	c. Movement of certain joints that decreases the angle between two adjoining bones.
_____ Flexion	d. Movement of the hand and forearm causing the palm to face downward or backward.
_____ Plantar flexion	
_____ Pronation	e. Movement of an extremity toward the axis of the body.
_____ Rotation	f. Movement of the hand and forearm that causes the palm to face upward or forward.
_____ Supination	
	g. Movement of certain joints that increases the angle between two adjoining bones.
	h. Movement of an extremity away from the midline of the body.
	i. Movement that causes the top of the foot to elevate or tilt upward.

3. Which of the following muscles are responsible for movement of the lower extremities? Select all that apply.

_____ Gluteus maximus

_____ Soleus

_____ Masseter

_____ Orbicularis oris

_____ Adductor longus

4. List the four most common types of arthritis.

5. Indicate whether each of the following statements is true or false.

a. _____ The skeletal muscles are under involuntary control.

b. _____ Rheumatoid arthritis affects an equal number of men and women.

c. _____ Children are often diagnosed with osteoarthritis.

6. Osteomyelitis is an infection of bone and/or bone marrow. What are the most common causes of osteomyelitis? (*Hint:* See page 143 in your textbook.)

7. What is the most common causative agent of osteomyelitis?

8. How is osteomyelitis treated?

Exercise 2

 CD-ROM Activity

 45 minutes

- Sign in to work at Pacific View Regional Hospital for Period of Care 1. (*Note:* If you are already in the virtual hospital from a previous exercise, click on **Leave the Floor** and then **Restart the Program** to get to the sign-in window.)
- From the Patient List, select Harry George (Room 401).
- Click on **Get Report** and read the Clinical Report.
- Click on **Go to Nurses' Station**; then click on **401** to go to the patient's room.
- Click on **Patient Care** and complete a head-to-toe assessment.

1. When you are assessing Harry George's affected extremity, which factors should you include in the assessment?

2. Harry George was admitted with a diagnosis of osteomyelitis. What findings support this diagnosis?

3. How does the affected extremity appear?

4. How does the assessment of the left (affected) leg differ from that of the right?

5. What other clinical manifestations may accompany a diagnosis of osteomyelitis?

6. How should the affected extremity be positioned?

→ • Click **Take Vital Signs** and review the information provided.

7. Discuss any findings in Harry George's vital signs that may indicate the presence of infection.

8. Which of the following diagnostic tests may be ordered to support a diagnosis of osteomyelitis? Select all that apply.

_____ MRI

_____ PET scan

_____ Bone scan

_____ X-rays

_____ Serum electrolytes

_____ Erythrocyte sedimentation rate

_____ Blood cultures

_____ Cultures of any drainage from open wounds

_____ Complete blood count

→ • Click **Chart** and then **401** to view Harry George's chart.
  • Click the **Laboratory Reports** and **Diagnostic Reports** tabs and review the information given.

9. What diagnostic tests were ordered for Harry George to support the diagnosis of osteomyelitis?

10. Which lab results support the diagnosis?

11. What findings were reported in the x-ray and bone scan?

→ • Click the **History and Physical** tab and review the report.

12. Based on your review of Harry George's medical and social history, what risk factors for osteomyelitis does he have?

13. What items in Harry George's assessment will be used to determine effectiveness of treatment?

➤ • Click the **Physician's Orders** tab and review the orders given.

14. What treatments have been ordered to manage Harry George's osteomyelitis?

15. To assist in the management of Harry George's care, what consultations has the physician ordered?

➤ • Click on **MAR** and then on tab **401**. Review the information given.

16. Which of the following medications have been prescribed to treat Harry George's osteomyelitis? Select all that apply.

_____ Gentamicin 20 mg IV

_____ Thiamine 100 mg PO/IM

_____ Glyburide 1.25 mg PO

_____ Cefotaxime 1 g IV

Care of the Patient Experiencing Comorbid Conditions (Musculoskeletal and Endocrine)

Reading Assignment: Care of the Patient with an Endocrine Disorder (Chapter 11)

Patient: Harry George, Room 401

Objectives:

1. Describe the functions of the endocrine system.
2. Discuss the dietary limitations of a patient with diabetes.
3. Describe the use of a sliding insulin scale.
4. Explain how type 1 and type 2 diabetes are similar and how they differ.
5. List disorders of the endocrine system.
6. Describe the tests used to assess for the presence of diabetes.

Exercise 1

 Writing Activity

30 minutes

1. The endocrine system functions alongside the _____ system to regulate many functions within the body, including metabolism, growth and development, and reproduction. The endocrine system communicates through the release of

   _____, which are chemical messengers that travel through the bloodstream to their target organs.

2. The _____ is considered the "master gland" of the endocrine system.

3. Match each of the following disorders of the pituitary gland with its correct description.

Disorder of the Pituitary Gland	**Description**
_____ Acromegaly	a. A transient or permanent metabolic disorder of the posterior pituitary in which ADH is deficient
_____ Gigantism	
_____ Dwarfism	b. A disorder in which the pituitary gland releases too much ADH and, in response, the kidneys reabsorb more water
_____ Diabetes insipidus	c. An overproduction of somatotropin in the adult
_____ Syndrome of inappropriate secretion of antidiuretic hormone (SIADH)	d. A condition in which there is a deficiency in growth hormone
	e. A condition that usually results from an over-secretion of growth hormone

4. What is diabetes?

5. How do the two types of diabetes mellitus differ? How are they similar? (*Hint:* See pages 542-543 in your textbook.)

6. The exact underlying cause of diabetes is unknown. There are, however, many theories about possible factors that may contribute to the development of diabetes. List several of those factors below.

7. Match each diagnostic test for diabetes with its function. (*Hint:* See Box 11-2 in your textbook.)

Test	**Function**
_____ Fasting blood sugar	a. This test is often used to determine whether a patient has type 1 or type 2 diabetes.
_____ Postprandial blood sugar	b. In this test, the fasting patient is provided with a carbohydrate solution to be ingested orally. Two hours after the administration, a blood sample will be drawn.
_____ Glycosylated hemoglobin	
_____ C peptide	
	c. This test consists of drawing a blood sample after the patient has fasted for an 8-hour period.
	d. This test measures the amount of glucose that has been incorporated into the body's hemoglobin. It reflects the patient's glucose elevations in the past 120 days.

8. Match each type of insulin with its correct onset of action after administration.

Type of Insulin	**Onset of Action After Administration**
_____ Humalog	a. 15-30 minutes
_____ Regular	b. 30-60 minutes
_____ NPH	c. 1-2 hours
_____ Lente (70/30)	d. 1-3 hours
_____ Lantus	e. 2-4 hours

9. Most available insulin is U/_____.

10. Indicate whether each of the following statements is true or false.

    a. _____ Urine testing is the recommended way of monitoring glucose levels in the IDDM patient.

    b. _____ Lantus should never be mixed with regular insulin.

    c. _____ Diabetics can choose between insulin or oral agents.

11. Insulin should be administered to the _____ tissue.

12. The site with the fastest rate of insulin absorption is the:
    a. abdomen.
    b. arms.
    c. thighs.
    d. buttocks.

13. The loss of fat deposits as a result of insulin administration is known as

    _____.

Exercise 2

 CD-ROM Activity

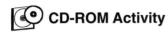 30 minutes

- Sign in to work at Pacific View Regional Hospital for Period of Care 1. (*Note:* If you are already in the virtual hospital from a previous exercise, click on **Leave the Floor** and then **Restart the Program** to get to the sign-in window.)
- From the Patient List, select Harry George (Room 401).
- Click on **Get Report** and read the Clinical Report.
- Click on **Go to Nurses' Station** and then click **Chart**.
- Click on **401** to view Harry George's chart.
- Click on the **Emergency Department** tab and review the information given.

1. What was Harry George's blood glucose upon his arrival at the emergency department?

2. What is the desired blood glucose level for a patient with diabetes?

3. Does Harry George have type 1 or type 2 diabetes mellitus?

4. What medication does Harry George take at home to control his diabetes?

5. How does this type of hypoglycemic medication work?

6. In addition to his daily scheduled medications to control his diabetes, Harry George has a sliding scale. Describe the use of a sliding scale.

7. _____ When Harry George's blood glucose is less than 150 mg/dL, his scheduled oral hypoglycemic medication will be held. (True or False)

8. The blood glucose of an ill patient with diabetes may require monitoring every _____ to

   _____ hours.

9. What impact might illness have on Harry George's blood glucose?

10. How does Harry George's diabetes affect his health status? For which additional complications might he be at risk because of his diabetes?

→ • Click **Return to Nurses' Station**; then click **401** to enter Harry George's room.
   • Click **Patient Care** and then **Nurse-Client Interactions**.
   • Select and view the video titled **0735: Symptom Management**. (*Note:* If this video is not available, check the virtual clock to see if enough time has elapsed. The video cannot be viewed before its specified time.)

11. What nonverbal behaviors are displayed by the patient, indicating a problem that needs to be addressed?

12. During the talk between Harry George and his "sitter," what needs and concerns are voiced?

13. What impact does the use of alcohol have on blood glucose level?

→ • Click **Chart** and then **401** to view Harry George's chart.
  • Click the **Physician's Orders** tab and review the orders.

14. What is the frequency of Harry George's blood glucose assessments?

15. What type of dietary management is being implemented?

16. Which of the following statements concerning Harry George's prescribed diet is correct?
    a. The diet will consist of three full meals per day to prevent snacking.
    b. The fat content should consist of no more than 30% of the caloric intake.
    c. 60% to 70 % of the calories in the diet should be from carbohydrates to ensure energy.
    d. Snacks should be avoided to reduce blood sugar fluctuations.

17. Harry George should be assessed for teaching needed in which areas?

  • Click **Return to Room 401**.
  • Click **Patient Care** and then **Nurse-Client Interactions**.
  • Select and view the video titled **0755: Disease Management**. (*Note:* If this video is not available, check the virtual clock to see if enough time has elapsed. The video cannot be viewed before its specified time.)

18. While talking with his sitter, Harry George continues to voice the need for his own "medication." What technique does the sitter attempt to employ to manage this request?

Developing a Plan of Care for a Patient with Osteomyelitis

Reading Assignment: Care of the Patient with a Musculoskeletal Disorder (Chapter 4)

Patient: Harry George, Room 401

Objectives:

1. Understand factors that affect pain management.
2. Identify nursing implications for the administration of narcotic analgesics.
3. Set priorities for the care of the patient with osteomyelitis.

Exercise 1

 CD-ROM Activity

 60 minutes

- Sign in to work at Pacific View Regional Hospital for Period of Care 2. (*Note:* If you are already in the virtual program from a previous exercise, click on **Leave the Floor** and then **Restart the Program** to get to the sign-in window.)
- From the Patient List, select Harry George (Room 401).
- Click on **Get Report** and read the Clinical Report.
- Click on **Go to Nurses' Station** and then **401** to enter Harry George's room.
- Read the **Initial Observations**.
- Click **Paitient Care** and complete a head-to-toe assessment.

1. What are the two primary priorities for Harry George's care at this time?

2. What elements of the assessment or the Clinical Report did you use to make this decision?

3. How has pain interfered with Harry George's recovery?

4. Is Harry George's pain a new problem or one that has been ongoing? Give a rationale for your response.

5. What nonpharmacologic interventions can be used to attempt to increase Harry George's level of comfort?

 • Click **Nurse-Client Interactions**.
   • Select and view the video titled **1120: Wound Management**. (*Note:* If this video is not available, check the virtual clock to see if enough time has elapsed. The video cannot be viewed before its specified time.)

6. What behaviors demonstrated by Harry George further support his report of pain and his level of anxiety?

• Now select and view the video titled **1125: Injury Prevention**.

7. During the interaction with his sitter, Harry George continues to appear nervous. His movements reflect jitteriness, and his extremities are trembling. To what can these behaviors be attributed?

• Click on **MAR** and then on tab **401** to review Harry George's MAR.

8. The physician has prescribed chlordiazepoxide hydrochloride. Other than anxiety, what is an indication for the use of this medication?

9. Which of the following nursing implications are indicated with the administration of chlordiazepoxide hydrochloride? Select all that apply.

   _____ Assess vital signs prior to administration.

   _____ Increase ambulation immediately after administration.

   _____ Administer cautiously in patients with liver impairments.

   _____ Institute safety precautions in regard to ambulation.

   _____ This medication may be used in patients who have recently ingested alcohol.

10. In addition to the chlordiazepoxide, what alternatives has the physician ordered to reduce Harry George's anxiety?

11. What factors will determine which of the medications should be given?

12. What medication has been ordered to manage Harry George's pain?

13. Does Harry George have any allergies that prevent him from being medicated with the drug prescribed? (*Hint:* Check his armband.)

14. Harry George's last dose of medication for pain was given at _____.

➡ • Click **Return to Room 401**. Then click the **Drug** icon.
  • Review the information provided for the medication you identified in question 12.

15. What elements of Harry George's medical/social history should be taken into consideration when administering this drug?

16. Are there any special administration precautions that must be observed when giving this medication IV push?

17. Are there any special considerations that must be taken when administering this drug in conjunction with the other medications currently in use?

18. Identify any safety measures that should be observed after administration of this medication.

19. Is it time for Harry George to be medicated again for pain?

→ • Click **Return to Room 401**. Then click **Take Vital Signs**.

20. What are Harry George's vital signs?

   BP:

   SpO$_2$:

   T:

   HR:

   RR:

   Pain:

21. What impact has Harry George's pain had on his vital signs?

22. Are Harry George's vital signs within acceptable limits to administer the drug that has been ordered to manage his pain?

23. If Harry George is unable to take his prescribed medications, what action(s) would be appropriate?

L E S S O N 4 _____

Postoperative Assessment

_____

👓 **Reading Assignment:** Care of the Surgical Patient (Chapter 2)
Care of the Patient with a Musculoskeletal Disorder (Chapter 4)

Patient: Clarence Hughes, Room 404

Objectives:

1. Define degenerative joint disease.
2. Identify the clinical signs and symptoms of degenerative joint disease.
3. Develop nursing diagnoses for the patient who has undergone joint replacement surgery.

Exercise 1

 Writing Activity

15 minutes

1. Which of the following populations are at an increased risk for developing degenerative joint disease? Select all that apply.

_____ Small-framed patients

_____ Obese patients

_____ Older patients

_____ Patients employed in occupations with activities that place joints in stressful positions

_____ Women of childbearing age

_____ Patients with diabetes

2. Degenerative joint disease is a nonsystemic, noninflammatory disorder of the joints that results in bone and joint degeneration. What are some signs and symptoms of degenerative joint disease?

3. _____ and _____ are two other names for degenerative joint disease.

4. What are some management techniques for degenerative joint disease?

5. What is arthroscopy?

Exercise 2

 CD-ROM Activity

 45 minutes

- Sign in to work at Pacific View Regional Hospital for Period of Care 1. (*Note:* If you are already in the virtual hospital from a previous exercise, click on **Leave the Floor** and then **Restart the Program** to get to the sign-in window.)
- From the Patient List, select Clarence Hughes (Room 404).
- Click **Get Report** and read the Clinical Report.
- Click on **Go to Nurses' Station** and then **404** to enter Clarence Hughes' room.
- Read the **Initial Observations**.
- Click **Chart** and then **404** to view Clarence Hughes' chart.
- Click the **History and Physical** tab and review the information given.

1. What signs and symptoms of degenerative joint disease has Clarence Hughes experienced?

2. What other methods of disease management did Clarence Hughes try prior to surgery?

 • Click **Return to Room 404**.
- Click **Clinical Alerts** and read the information given.
- Now click **Patient Care** and complete a head-to-toe assessment.

3. _____ Findings from Clarence Hughes' physical assessment warrant physician notification. (True or False)

4. What are the two most important priorities for care at this time?

5. Develop two individualized nursing diagnoses for this patient.

6. Why are these issues most important to the successful management of Clarence Hughes' care?

7. Are there any abnormal findings in the abdominal assessment?

→ • Click **MAR** and then tab **404** to review Clarence Hughes' record.

8. What medication options are available to manage Clarence Hughes' pain?

→ • Click **Return to Room 404**.
   • Click the **Drug** icon and review the pain medication(s) prescribed for Clarence Hughes.

9. Does Clarence Hughes have any contraindications for the pain medication(s) you identified in question 8?

10. What side effects can be anticipated with administration of the medication(s)?

11. Discuss any safety precautions that may need to be instituted with use of the medication(s).

12. Discuss any special monitoring that will be needed with the administration of the medication(s).

13. What regularly scheduled medication has been ordered to reduce the patient's constipation? What is the mechanism of action for this medication?

14. What prn medications have been ordered to reduce constipation? How do these medications work?

→ • Click **Return to Room 404**.
 • Click **Chart** and then **404** to view Clarence Hughes' chart.
 • Click the **Physician's Notes** tab.

15. What are the physician's plans concerning Clarence Hughes' discharge?

→ • Click the **Consultations** tab.

16. What consultations have been ordered for Clarence Hughes? What is the purpose of these consultations?

→ • Click the **Patient Education** tab.

17. What are Clarence Hughes' educational needs?

LESSON 5

Postoperative Complications

👓 **Reading Assignment:** Care of the Surgical Patient (Chapter 2)

Care of the Patient with a Respiratory Disorder (Chapter 9)

Patient: Clarence Hughes, Room 404

Objectives:

1. Identify potential postoperative complications.
2. Recognize clinical manifestations associated with the development of postoperative complications.
3. Review the management/treatment of a postoperative complication involving the respiratory system.

Exercise 1

Writing Activity

 15 minutes

1. List several potential postoperative complications.

2. The collapse of lung tissue, which results in the lack of adequate exchange of oxygen and

   carbon dioxide, is known as _____.

Hint: Refer to pages 446-448 in your textbook for the next several questions.

3. What is a pulmonary embolism?

4. When you are assessing the patient for a pulmonary embolism, which of the following manifestations can be anticipated? Select all that apply.

   _____ Dull and achy pain

   _____ Pain often described as sharp

   _____ Pain that radiates to the back and neck

   _____ Nonradiating pain

   _____ Dyspnea

   _____ Reduced respiratory rate

   _____ Increased respiratory rate

   _____ Increased pain with inspiration

5. During the initial period after onset and subsequent diagnosis of pulmonary embolism, which of the following treatments can be anticipated? Select all that apply.

_____ Oxygen

_____ Oral anticoagulants

_____ Intramuscular antibiotics

_____ Intravenous anticoagulants

_____ Hydration

6. How is a pulmonary embolism managed?

7. What is the prognosis for a patient who develops a pulmonary embolism?

8. What is a ventilation perfusion scan?

Exercise 2

  CD-ROM Activity

 30 minutes

- Sign in to work at Pacific View Regional Hospital for Period of Care 2. (*Note:* If you are already in the virtual hospital from a previous exercise, click on **Leave the Floor** and then **Restart the Program** to get to the sign-in window.)
- From the Patient List, select Clarence Hughes (Room 404).
- Click on **Get Report** and read the Clinical Report.

1. Are there any abnormal observations in the change-of-shift report?

2. Review the vital signs recorded in the change-of-shift report. Are they normal?

→ • Click **Go to Nurses' Station** and then **404** to enter the patient's room.
- Read the **Initial Observation**.
- Click **Clinical Alerts** and read the information provided.

3. Which clinical findings indicate a problem?

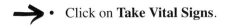 • Click on **Take Vital Signs**.

4. What are Clarence Hughes' current vital signs?

BP:

T:

HR:

RR:

5. Are any of the above results abnormal? If so, which?

6. What is Clarence Hughes' current oxygen saturation? Is this a normal value? If not, how should it be managed?

 • Click **Patient Care** and then **Nurse-Client Interactions**.
 • Select and view the video titled **1115: Interventions—Airway**. (*Note:* If this video is unavailable, check the virtual clock to see if enough time has elapsed. The video cannot be viewed until its specified time.)

7. What behavioral cues being demonstrated by Clarence Hughes indicate a problem?

8. What should be the nurse's interventions (in priority order)?

➤ • Click **Physical Assessment** and complete a head-to-toe assessment.

9. Are there any significant findings identified in the integumentary assessment?

10. Are there any significant findings identified in the respiratory assessment?

➤ • Click **Chart** and then **404** to view Clarence Hughes' chart.
   • Click the **Physician's Orders** tab and review the orders listed for 1120 on Wednesday.

11. What tests and interventions has the physician ordered?

12. The degree of anxiety is often directly tied to the amount of _____ hunger being experienced by the patient.

• Click **Return to Room 404**.
 • Click **Patient Care** and then **Nurse-Client Interactions**.
 • Select and view the video titled **1135: Change in Patient Condition**. (*Note:* If this video is not available, check the virtual clock to see if enough time has elapsed. The video cannot be viewed before its specified time.)

13. Now that the initial crisis has passed, what are the nurse's priorities concerning the family members?

Exercise 3

 CD-ROM Activity

15 minutes

- Sign in to work at Pacific View Regional Hospital for Period of Care 3. (*Note:* If you are already in the virtual hospital from the previous exercise, click on **Leave the Floor** and then on **Restart the Program** to get to the sign-in window.)
- From the Patient List, select Clarence Hughes (Room 404).
- Click on **Get Report** and read the Clinical Report.

1. Give the results for each of the tests listed below.

   Arterial blood gas:

   Chest x-ray:

   Ventilation perfusion scan:

   Doppler study:

 - Click **Go to Nurses' Station**.
- Click **404** to enter Clarence Hughes' room.
- Read the **Initial Observations**.
- Click and review the **Clinical Alerts**.

2. What changes are noted in the patient's demeanor and clinical manifestations?

 - Click **Take Vital Signs** and review the results.

3. What is the significance of the increasing SO_2 level?

• Click **Chart** and then **404** to review Clarence Hughes' chart.
  • Click the **Physician's Orders** tab and review the information given.

4. What medication has been ordered to manage Clarence Hughes' condition? Describe the administration of this medication.

5. What are the method of action and the purpose for the administration of this medication?

6. What is the classification of this medication?

7. During therapy with the medication identified in question 4, which of the following laboratory tests is most important to monitor?
  a. PTT
  b. Hgb
  c. Hct
  d. WBC
  e. ESR

Care of the Patient with Pneumonia

👓 **Reading Assignment:** Care of the Patient with a Respiratory Disorder (Chapter 9)

Patient: Patricia Newman, Room 406

Objectives:

1. Define pneumonia.
2. Identify the potential causes of pneumonia.
3. Identify the populations at risk for pneumonia.
4. Discuss nursing care for the patient with pneumonia.

Exercise 1

Writing Activity

  30 minutes

1. What is pneumonia?

2. Infants and the _____ are most susceptible to pneumonia.

3. What factors could make people more susceptible to pneumonia?

4. Which of the following may contribute to the development of pneumonia? Select all that apply.

_____ Overuse of steroid medications

_____ Infection

_____ Hyperventilation

_____ Inadequate ventilation

_____ Aspiration

_____ Poor nutritional habits

5. Match the columns below to show the correct order of pathologic occurrences associated with the development of pneumonia. (*Hint:* See page 434 in your textbook.)

Disease Process	**Order of Occurrence**
_____ The respiratory tract develops inflammation and localized edema.	a. First
	b. Second
_____ The exchange of oxygen and carbon dioxide becomes increasingly reduced.	c. Third
_____ Secretions begin to accumulate and are not able to be moved by the cilia in the lungs.	d. Fourth
_____ Retained secretions become infected.	

6. When caring for a patient diagnosed with pneumonia, which of the following nursing interventions are appropriate? Select all that apply.

_____ Keep patient on complete bedrest.

_____ Encourage deep breathing and coughing activities.

_____ Initiate exercise training.

_____ Provide patient education aimed as reducing the spread of infection.

_____ Restrict protein intake.

_____ Monitor vital signs and pulmonary status.

_____ Provide information concerning the prescribed medication therapy.

_____ Encourage fluid intake if not contraindicated by patient's coexisting conditions.

7. What is the typical prognosis for a patient with pneumonia?

8. When assisting the patient with pneumonia to plan meals, which of the following dietary recommendations should be implemented? (*Hint:* See page 436 in your textbook.)
   a. Three large balanced meals each day will be best to provide the needed nutrients.
   b. The diet should include at least 3000 calories per day.
   c. Protein and sodium are indicated.
   d. The diet should consist of at least 1500 calories each day.

9. What is the purpose of the above dietary intervention?

Exercise 2

  CD-ROM Activity

45 minutes

- Sign in to work at Pacific View Regional Hospital for Period of Care 1. (*Note:* If you are already in the virtual hospital from a previous exercise, click on **Leave the Floor** and **Restart the Program** to get to the sign-in window.)
- From the Patient List, select Patricia Newman (Room 406).
- Click on **Get Report** and read the Clinical Report.
- Click on **Go to Nurses' Station** then on **406** to view Patricia Newman's chart.
- Click the **Emergency Department** tab and review the information given.

1. What were the findings of the Initial Assessment in the emergency department?

2. Discuss any abnormal findings in her respiratory system assessment.

3. Find the vital sign results on the ED record and discuss the significance of these findings.

4. What are the primary and secondary admitting diagnoses?

LESSON 6—CARE OF THE PATIENT WITH PNEUMONIA   **85**

5. Listed below are laboratory tests ordered for Patricia Newman while in the emergency department. Match each laboratory test with its reason for being ordered.

Laboratory Test	**Reason It Was Ordered**
_____ Sputum Gram stain	a. Ordered to provide information about the potential presence of infection and the body's response
_____ Arterial blood gases	b. Ordered to identify specific pathogens in a specimen
_____ Complete blood count	c. Ordered to identify the specific pathogens and determine which medications therapies will be most effective
_____ Culture and sensitivity	
_____ Erythrocyte sedimentation rate	d. Ordered to identify the presence and degree of inflammation in the body
	e. Ordered to definitely evaluate the oxygen levels in the body

6. What is the purpose of the x-ray ordered for this patient?

→ • Click **Return to Room 406** and review the **Initial Observations**.

7. Discuss the significance of the oxygen saturation and the patient's removal of the nasal cannula.

8. _____ Patricia Newman's arterial blood gas results are within normal limits. (True or False)

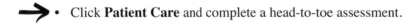 • Click **Take Vital Signs** and review the results provided.

9. What are the patient's current vital signs, including oxygen saturation and pain level?

   BP:

   SpO$_2$:

   T:

   HR:

   RR:

   Pain:

10. What is the significance of these findings?

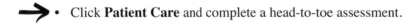 • Click **Patient Care** and complete a head-to-toe assessment.

11. What assessment findings support the admitting diagnosis of pneumonia?

→ • Click **MAR** and then tab **406** to review the medications ordered for Patricia Newman.

12. The following drugs have been ordered to manage Patricia Newman's pneumonia. Match each drug with its correct classification.

Drug	Classification
_____ Acetaminophen	a. Antipyretic
_____ Cefotan	b. Antiinflammatory
_____ Ipratropium	c. Antibiotic
	d. Bronchodilator
	e. Corticosteroid

→ • Click **Return to Room 406**.
   • Click **Chart** and then **406** to view Patricia Newman's chart.
   • Click the **Laboratory Reports** tab and review the information given.

13. Discuss the significance of the culture and sensitivity test results.

14. Review and discuss the findings of the complete blood count test.

→ • Click the **Diagnostic Reports** tab and review the report.

15. Review the findings of the chest x-ray in relation to the diagnosis of pneumonia.

16. Which clinical manifestations will reflect positive impact of treatments?

Care of the Patient Experiencing Comorbid Conditions (Musculoskeletal and Respiratory)

Reading Assignment: Care of the Patient with a Musculoskeletal Disorder (Chapter 4)
Care of the Patient with a Cardiovascular or a Peripheral
Vascular Disorder (Chapter 8)
Care of the Patient with a Respiratory Disorder (Chapter 9)

Patient: Patricia Newman, Room 406

Objectives:

1. Identify significant findings in a patient's medical history.
2. Identify significant findings in a patient's social history.
3. Discuss the pathophysiology, risk factors, and management of hypertension.
4. Discuss the pathophysiology, risk factors, and management of osteoporosis.
5. Discuss the pathophysiology, risk factors, and management of emphysema.
6. Identify important issues in caring for the patient with comorbid conditions.

Exercise 1

 Writing Activity

30 minutes

1. Hypertension occurs when blood pressure is sustained at systolic readings above

   _____ and/or diastolic readings greater than _____.

2. Which of the following risk factors are associated with hypertension? Select all that apply.

   _____ Obesity

   _____ Genetic factors

   _____ Sedentary lifestyle

   _____ Diabetes

   _____ Asthma

   _____ Increased sodium intake

   _____ Excessive alcohol ingestion

3. List three medical management options for the treatment of hypertension.

4. What is emphysema?

5. What risk factors are associated with emphysema?

6. List several clinical manifestations of emphysema. (*Hint:* See page 451 in your textbook.)

7. What are the management options for the patient with emphysema?

8. What is the usual prognosis for a patient diagnosed with emphysema?

9. Osteoporosis is a disease characterized by the reduction in _____.

10. Which of the following are at high risk for the development of osteoporosis? Select all that apply. (*Hint:* See page 140 in your textbook.)

_____ Women

_____ Large-framed individuals

_____ Smokers

_____ Those with sedentary lifestyles

_____ People taking supplements to increase calcium intake

_____ Users of steroids

_____ Immobilized individuals

_____ Postmenopausal women

_____ African Americans

11. What areas of the body are most affected by osteoporosis?

12. List several clinical manifestations associated with osteoporosis.

13. When planning the care of a patient diagnosed with osteoporosis, which of the following may be included? Select all that apply.

_____ Exercise

_____ Restricted levels of activity

_____ Increased calcium intake/supplements

_____ Estrogen therapy

_____ Reduced protein intake

14. To plan a diet high in calcium, which of the following should be included?
    a. Yellow vegetables
    b. Tomatoes
    c. Dates and legumes
    d. Green leafy vegetables

15. The coexistence of osteoporosis, emphysema, and hypertension presents what unique problems for Patricia Newman?

Exercise 2

  CD-ROM Activity

45 minutes

- Sign in to work at Pacific View Regional Hospital for Period of Care 4. (*Note:* If you are already in the virtual hospital from a previous exercise, click on **Leave the Floor** and **Restart the Program** to get to the sign-in window.)
- From the Patient List, select Patricia Newman (Room 406).
- Click on **Get Report** and read the Clinical Report.
- Click on **Go to Nurses' Station** and then on **Chart**.
- Click on **406** to view Patricia Newman's chart.
- Click the **History and Physical** tab and review the information given.

1. What significant medical issues are in Patricia Newman's medical history?

2. Does the patient have any surgeries in her medical history?

3. Describe Patricia Newman's social history.

➡ • Click the **Nursing Admission** tab and review the information given.

4. What factors in Patricia Newman's history are related to a diagnosis of emphysema?

5. How is her recurring history of pneumonia related to her emphysema?

6. What factors in her history support a diagnosis of osteoporosis?

➡ • Click **Return to Nurses' Station**.
   • Click **MAR** and then tab **406** to view the medications ordered for Patricia Newman.

7. What medications have been prescribed to manage Patricia Newman's hypertension?

8. Describe the mode of action for each of the medications you identified in question 7.

9. When you are planning care for the patient being treated with the above medications, which of the following laboratory tests must be monitored?
   a. Serum sodium levels
   b. Serum potassium levels
   c. Erythrocyte sedimentation rate
   d. Complete blood count results

10. What medications have been ordered to manage Patricia Newman's emphysema?

11. What medication has been prescribed to manage Patricia Newman's osteoporosis?

12. When you are administering the medication ordered to manage osteoporosis, which of the following nursing implications is indicated? Select all that apply.

   _____ Administer medication 15–30 minutes before eating.

   _____ Administer medication with juice to improve absorption.

   _____ Administer medication 30–60 minutes after eating.

   _____ Monitor blood pressure.

   _____ Administer with foods high in fiber.

Prioritizing Care for a Patient with a Pulmonary Disorder

Reading Assignment: Care of the Patient with a Respiratory Disorder (Chapter 9)

Patient: Patricia Newman, Room 406

Objectives:

1. Identify the primary patient education teaching goals for the patient experiencing a pulmonary disorder.
2. Discuss the appropriate service consultations for a patient experiencing a pulmonary disorder.
3. Determine the impact of personal/social factors in the patient's recovery period.
4. Develop priorities for the patient during hospitalization and in preparation for discharge.

Exercise 1

 Writing Activity

🕐 30 minutes

1. Which of the following are characteristics associated with emphysema? Select all that apply.

    _____ Emphysema affects both men and women.

    _____ Emphysema symptoms typically begin to manifest while the patient is in the mid-to late 30s.

    _____ The disorder is characterized by changes in the alveolar walls and capillaries.

    _____ Disability often results in patients diagnosed with emphysema between ages 50 and 60 years.

    _____ Heredity may play a role in the development of emphysema.

2. When diagnostic tests are ordered to confirm the presence of emphysema, which of the following diagnostic tests should be anticipated? Select all that apply.

    _____ Thoracentesis

    _____ Arterial blood gases

    _____ Complete blood cell count

    _____ Chest x-ray

    _____ Bronchoscopy

    _____ Pulse oximetry

3. When caring for a patient diagnosed with emphysema, the nurse should anticipate which of the following results for a pulmonary function test?
   a. Reduced residual volume
   b. Reduced airway resistance
   c. Increased ventilatory response
   d. Increased residual volume

4. The complete blood cell count will reflect which of the following results in a patient diagnosed with emphysema?
   a. Reduced erythrocyte count
   b. Elevated erythrocyte count
   c. Elevated erythrocyte count and reduced hemoglobin
   d. Reduced erythrocyte count and elevated hemoglobin

5. In the patient who is experiencing emphysema, which of the following best reflects the anticipated pulmonary function tests?
   a. Increased PaO_2
   b. Decreased PaO_2
   c. Reduced residual volume
   d. Increased total lung capacity

6. Describe the disease process associated with emphysema.

7. Indicate whether each of the following statements is true or false.

    a. _____ An inherited form of emphysema is due to an oversecretion of a liver protein known as ATT.

    b. _____ Hypercapnia does not develop until the later stages of emphysema.

8. Discuss the use of exercise in the care and management of the patient diagnosed with emphysema.

9. _____ is an abnormal cardiac condition characterized by hypertrophy of the right ventricle of the heart due to hypertension of the pulmonary circulation.

10. The complete blood cell count will demonstrate which of the following characteristics in the patient with emphysema?
    a. The erythrocyte level will be within normal limits.
    b. The erythrocyte count will be elevated, and the hematocrit levels will be reduced.
    c. The erythrocytes, hematocrit, and hemoglobin values will be elevated.
    d. The erythrocyte count will be reduced, and the hematocrit and hemoglobin levels will be elevated.

Exercise 2

 CD-ROM Activity

 30 minutes

- Sign in to work at Pacific View Regional Hospital for Period of Care 3. (*Note:* If you are already in the virtual hospital from a previous exercise, click on **Leave the Floor** and **Restart the Program** to get to the sign-in window.)
- From the Patient List, select Patricia Newman (Room 406).
- Click on **Get Report** and read the Clinical Report.
- Click on **Go to Nurses' Station** and then on **406** to enter the patient's room.
- Read the **Initial Observations**.
- Click **Patient Care** and then **Nurse-Client Interactions**.
- Select and view the video titled **1500: Discharge Planning**. (*Note:* If this video is not available, check the virtual clock to see if enough time has elapsed. The video cannot be viewed before its specified time.)

1. Discuss Patricia Newman's demeanor during the nurse-client interaction.

2. What appear to be the patient's biggest concerns in the nurse-client interaction?

→ • Click **Physical Assessment** and complete a head-to-toe assessment.

3. What evidence suggests that Patricia Newman's condition is improving?

4. Are there any assessment findings that have a potentially negative implication for Patricia Newman's discharge to home?

5. As you develop Patricia Newman's plan of care, which of the following are priorities at this time? Select all that apply.

_____ Dietary counseling

_____ Preparation for discharge

_____ Referrals for smoking cessation programs

_____ Requesting a consultation with physical therapy

_____ Requesting a consultation with social services

6. Develop three nursing diagnoses for Patricia Newman.

• Click **Chart** and then **406** to view Patricia Newman's chart.
• Click the **Nursing Admission** tab and review the information given.

7. Identify Patricia Newman's social concerns.

8. Which of the following statements accurately reflects an aspect of the patient's needs?
   a. She has numerous friends and family members available to provide assistance.
   b. She appears self-sufficient and needs little outside help.
   c. She is somewhat socially isolated.
   d. Her significant other will be available as needed for assistance after discharge.

9. Discuss the implications of these social concerns on the nurse's plan of care for Patricia Newman.

→ • Click the **Patient Education** tab and review the information given.

10. As Patricia Newman prepares to go home, which of the following are educational goals for her discharge? Select all that apply.

_____ Correct use of MDI and peak flow meter

_____ Understanding rationale for and performance of pursed-lip breathing and effective cough technique

_____ The need to be sedentary to avoid further complications

_____ Understanding of and compliance with prescribed medication therapy

_____ Compliance with progressive activity/exercise goals

11. Considering Patricia Newman's social and financial history, which of the goals may be a challenge for her to meet?

12. To assist Patricia Newman in complying with her discharge plans, consultations/referrals

will be needed with _____ and

_____ programs.

→ • Click the **Physician's Orders** tab.

13. What consultations have been ordered for Patricia Newman during this hospitalization?

LESSON **9**

Care of the Patient Experiencing Exacerbation of an Asthmatic Condition

≈ **Reading Assignment:** Care of the Patient with a Respiratory Disorder (Chapter 9)

Patient: Jacquline Catanazaro, Room 402

Objectives:

1. Define asthma.
2. Identify factors that contribute to an asthmatic episode.
3. Report assessment findings consistent with an exacerbation of asthma.
4. Discuss the impact of emotional distress on the respiratory system.

Exercise 1

 Writing Activity

15 minutes

1. What is asthma?

2. Which of the following events can trigger an asthmatic episode? Select all that apply.

   _____ Hormone levels

   _____ Mental and physical fatigue

   _____ Emotional factors

   _____ Environmental exposures

   _____ Electrolyte imbalances

3. List the clinical manifestations of mild asthma.

4. Review the signs and symptoms associated with an acute asthmatic attack.

5. When an asthmatic condition is suspected, which of the following diagnostic tests will confirm a diagnosis? Select all that apply.

_____ Complete blood count

_____ Serum electrolyte levels

_____ Arterial blood gas

_____ Pulmonary function tests

_____ Sputum cultures

6. What is the prognosis for asthma?

7. Which of the following statements is correct concerning the impact of oxygen saturation levels on the body's functioning?
   a. Saturation rates of 95% to 100% are needed to replenish oxygen in the plasma.
   b. Saturation rates below 90% affect the ability of hemoglobin to feed oxygen to the plasma.
   c. Saturation levels below 70% are considered life-threatening.
   d. Saturation levels below 85% warrant contacting the physician.

Exercise 2

 CD-ROM Activity

 45 minutes

- Sign in to work at Pacific View Regional Hospital for Period of Care 1. (*Note:* If you are already in the virtual hospital from a previous exercise, click on **Leave the Floor** and **Restart the Program** to get to the sign-in window.)
- From the Patient List, select Jacquline Catanazaro (Room 402).
- Click on **Get Report** and read the Clinical Report.
- Click on **Go to Nurses' Station**.
- Click **Chart** and then **402** to view Jacquline Catanazaro's chart.
- Click the **Emergency Department** tab and review the information given.

   1. Review the admitting vital signs. What is the significance of the findings?

   2. What is the primary admitting diagnosis?

 • Click **Return to Nurses' Station** and then **402**.
- Read the **Initial Observations**.
- Click **Take Vital Signs** and review the results provided.
- Click **Clinical Alerts** and read the report.

   3. Jacquline Catanazaro is demonstrating extreme agitation. What is the impact of these behaviors on her health status?

4. _____   When you are using the pulse oximeter, the probe should be placed over a pulsating vascular bed. (True or False)

5. When you are performing a pulse oximeter reading for the patient, which of the following sites is appropriate? Select all that apply.

_____ Ear lobe

_____ Bridge of the nose

_____ Tip of the nose

_____ Finger

_____ Toe

→ • Click **Patient Care** and then **Nurse-Client Interactions**.

• Select and view the video titled **0730: Intervention—Airway**. (*Note:* If this video is not available, check the virtual clock to see if enough time has elapsed. The video cannot be viewed before its specified time.)

6. Jacquline Catanazaro is experiencing an acute asthma attack. What has been planned to manage the onset?

7. What will the arterial blood gases determine?

→ • Click **Physical Assessment** and complete a head-to-toe assessment.

8. What respiratory system findings in Jacquline Catanazaro's assessment are consistent with an exacerbation of asthma?

9. Are there any other significant system findings?

→ • Click **Chart** and then **402** to view Jacquline Catanazaro's chart.
   • Click the **Physician's Orders** tab and note the admission orders for Monday at 1600.
   • Click **Return to Room 402** and then click the **Drug** icon.
   • Review the information for the drugs that have been prescribed for Jacquline Catanazaro.

10. What are the doses and routes of administration for each medication ordered to manage Jacquline Catanazaro's respiratory condition?

   a. Beclomethasone:

   b. Albuterol:

   c. Ipratropium bromide:

11. Match each prescribed medication with its correct mode of action.

Medication	Mode of Action
_____ Beclomethasone	a. Relief of bronchospasms
_____ Albuterol	b. Reduction of bronchial inflammation
_____ Ipratropium bromide	c. Control of secretions

12. When providing patient education concerning the use of beclomethasone, the nurse should tell the patient that which of the following side effects may occur?
    a. Throat irritation
    b. Productive cough
    c. Increased pulmonary secretions
    d. Skin rash
    e. Activity intolerance

 • Click **Return to Room 402**.
    • Click **Chart** and then **402**.
    • Click the **Physician's Orders** tab and review the orders for Monday at 1600.

13. What tests and/or assessments will be used to monitor Jacquline Catanazaro's respiratory status?

14. List several clinical manifestations that will indicate improvement in the patient's condition.

 • Click **Return to Room 402**.
    • Click **Patient Care** and then **Nurse-Client Interactions**.
    • Select and view the video titled **0800: Managing Altered Perceptions**. (*Note:* If this video is not available, check the virtual clock to see if enough time has elapsed. The video cannot be viewed before its specified time.)

15. What medication has been ordered for Jacquline Catanazaro?

16. What are the classification and mode of action for this medication?

Developing a Plan of Care for the Asthmatic Patient with Psychological Complications

⌒ᴑᴑᴑ **Reading Assignment:** Care of the Patient with a Respiratory Disorder (Chapter 9)

Patient: Jacquline Catanazaro, Room 402

Objectives:

1. Evaluate the impact of the patient's social history on anticipated compliance after discharge.
2. Identify the elements to be incorporated into the teaching plan in preparation for discharge.
3. Develop nursing diagnoses for the patient experiencing coexisting psychological and physiological conditions.

Exercise 1

Writing Activity

15 minutes

1. _____ is a severe asthmatic attack that fails to respond to the normal treatment plan.

2. Extrinsic factors associated with an asthmatic attack include which of the following? Select all that apply.

   _____ Infection

   _____ Dust

   _____ Pollen

   _____ Exercise

   _____ Foods

3. Indicate whether each of the following statements is true or false.

   a. _____ Encouraging the patient experiencing an asthma attack to lean back will aid in breathing ability.

   b. _____ The death rate for asthma has been declining over the past 10 years because of the advances in pharmacologic therapies.

4. A complete blood cell count will reflect an elevation in which of the following in the patient experiencing an asthma attack?
   a. Eosinophils
   b. Platelets
   c. Red blood cells
   d. Monocytes

5. Which of the following is considered an acceptable range for a therapeutic level of theophylline?
   a. 35-45 mcg/mL
   b. Less than 4 mcg/mL
   c. 10-20 mcg/mL
   d. Greater than 50 mcg/mL

6. A _____ should be obtained to rule out a secondary infection.

7. Which of the following statements concerning asthma is true?
   a. Air tubes narrow as a result of swollen tissues and excessive mucus production.
   b. There is edema of respiratory mucosa and excessive mucous production, which obstructs airways.
   c. The walls of the alveoli are torn and cannot be repaired.
   d. The bronchioles are scarred and unable to expand.

8. Match each of the following drugs with its correct classification. (*Hint:* See page 458 in your textbook.)

Drug	**Classification**
_____ Serevent	a. Corticosteroid
_____ Flovent	b. Long-acting beta receptor agonist
_____ Adrenalin	c. Short-acting beta receptor agonist
_____ Proventil	d. Bronchodilator

Exercise 2

 CD-ROM Activity

 45 minutes

- Sign in to work at Pacific View Regional Hospital for Period of Care 2. (*Note:* If you are already in the Virtual Hospital from a previous exercise, click on **Leave the Floor** and **Restart the Program** to get to the sign-in window.)
- From the Patient List, select Jacquline Catanazaro (Room 402).
- Click on **Get Report** and read the Clinical Report.

1. Describe the psychological behaviors documented in the two change-of-shift reports.

2. How do these psychological behaviors affect Jacquline Catanazaro's condition?

 • Click **Go to Nurses' Station** and then **402**.
- Read the **Initial Observations**.
- Click **Take Vital Signs** and review the information given.
- Click **Patient Care** and complete a head-to-toe assessment.
- Next, click **Nurse-Client Interactions**.
- Select and view the video titled **1115: Assessment—Readiness to Learn**. (*Note:* If this video is not available, check the virtual clock to see if enough time has elapsed. The video cannot be viewed until its specified time.)

3. What is the focus of the nurse-client interaction?

4. Do social supports appear to be available for Jacquline Catanazaro?

5. What are the priorities of care associated with Jacquline Catanazaro's psychosocial needs?

6. What are the priorities of care associated with Jacquline Catanazaro's physiological needs?

→ • Click **Chart** and then **402** to view Jacquline Catanazaro's chart.
  • Click the **History and Physical** tab and review the information given.

7. List some significant issues identified in Jacquline Catanazaro's medical history.

8. List several significant issues identified in Jacquline Catanazaro's social history.

9. Describe the interrelationships among the medical and social elements in Jacquline Catanazaro's history.

10. What factors in Jacquline Catanazaro's medical history will significantly affect her discharge?

11. How does Jacquline Catanazaro's mental health affect her physical health?

➤ • Click the **Consultations** tab and review the information given.

12. Discuss the plan identified in the Psychiatric Consult report.

→ • Click the **Patient Education** tab and review the education goals listed.

13. What are the educational goals identified?

14. Who should be included in the teaching plan for Jacquline Catanazaro?

15. Develop two nursing diagnoses for the patient at this point in her care.

11

Care and Treatment of the Patient with Complications of Cancer

/OR **Reading Assignment:** Care of the Patient with Cancer (Chapter 17)

Patient: Pablo Rodriguez, Room 405

Objectives:

1. Discuss complications associated with cancer.
2. Discuss the management of the patient experiencing dehydration secondary to chemotherapy.
3. Prioritize the problems of the patient experiencing complications of cancer.
4. Evaluate abnormal laboratory findings.

Exercise 1

Writing Activity

15 minutes

- Sign in to work at Pacific View Regional Hospital for Period of Care 2. (*Note:* If you are already in the virtual hospital from a previous exercise, click on **Leave the Floor** and then **Restart the Program** to get to the sign-in window.)
- From the Patient List, select Pablo Rodriguez (Room 405).
- Click **Get Report** and read the **Clinical Report**.
- Click **Go to Nurses' Station** and then **405** to view Pablo Rodriguez's chart.
- Click the **Emergency Department** tab and review the information given.

1. What are the four priorities identified in the change-of-shift report?

2. Why was Pablo Rodriguez admitted to the hospital?

3. What has caused this condition?

4. What findings support this diagnosis?

5. How was his condition initially managed in the emergency department?

6. What types of interventions (nursing and medical) may be implemented to manage his care?

7. What should be monitored to determine the degree of dehydration?

8. What are the primary goals for this hospitalization?

→ • Click the **History and Physical** tab and read the report.

9. List the impressions identified in the History and Physical.

Exercise 2

 CD-ROM Activity

 30 minutes

- Sign in to work at Pacific View Regional Hospital for Period of Care 2. (*Note:* If you are already in the virtual hospital from a previous exercise, click on **Leave the Floor** and **Restart the Program** to get to the sign-in window.)
- From the Patient List, select Pablo Rodriguez (Room 405).
- Click **Go to Nurses' Station**
- Click **405** to enter Pablo Rodriguez's room.
- Read the **Initial Observations**.
- Click **Take Vital Signs** and then **Clinical Alerts** and review the information given.
- Read the **Initial Observations.**
- Click **Patient Care** and complete a head-to-toe assessment.

1. What current assessment findings support the diagnosis of dehydration?

- Click **Chart** and then **405** to view Pablo Rodriguez's chart.
- Click the **Physician's Orders** tab and review the orders since Tuesday at 2300.

2. Which medications have been ordered to manage Pablo Rodriguez's nausea?

- Click **Return to Room 405** and then click the **Drug** icon.
- Review the medications you identified in the previous question.

3. To what drug classification does ondansetron hydrochloride belong?

4. What side effects of ondansetron could be problematic, considering Pablo Rodriguez's health concerns?

5. What is metoclopramide's mechanism of action?

 • Click **Return to Room 405**.
   • Click **Chart** and then **405** to view Pablo Rodriguez's chart.
   • Click the **Laboratory Reports** tab and review the report given.

6. Review and discuss any significant findings in the CBC results.

7. What signs and symptoms may be attributed to the CBC results?

8. Are there any significant findings in the electrolyte profile?

9. Identify two nursing diagnoses related to Pablo Rodriguez's primary admitting diagnosis.

Exercise 3

 CD-ROM Activity

 30 minutes

- Sign in to work at Pacific View Regional Hospital for Period of Care 2. (*Note:* If you are already in the virtual hospital from a previous exercise, click on **Leave the Floor** and then **Restart the Program** to get to the sign-in window.)
- From the Patient List, select Pablo Rodriguez (Room 405).
- Click **Get Report** and read the **Clinical Report**.
- Click **Go to Nurses' Station** and then **405** to enter Pablo Rodriguez's room.
- Click **Take Vital Signs** and review the information given.

1. How does Pablo Rodriguez rate his pain?

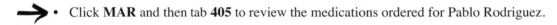 • Click **MAR** and then tab **405** to review the medications ordered for Pablo Rodriguez.

2. What medications have been ordered to manage Pablo Rodriguez's pain?

3. What is the advantage of this type of dosing?

4. List some opioids that may be prescribed to manage the pain associated with advanced cancer.

5. What side effects are associated with opioid administration?

6. List several nonopioid medications that can be administered to reduce mild to moderate pain associated with cancer.

7. Discuss medication scheduling techniques that effectively manage pain.

8. As previously stated, Pablo Rodriguez has been experiencing anxiety. Discuss the relationship between pain and anxiety.

9. In addition to medication therapy, what other interventions may be used to manage pain?

10. What factors may influence a patient's perception of and/or reaction to pain?

 • Click **Return to Room 405**.
   • Click **Patient Care** and then **Nurse-Client Interactions**.
   • Select and view the video titled **1130: Family Interaction**. (*Note:* If this video is not available, check the virtual clock to see if enough time has elapsed. The video cannot be viewed until its specified time.)

11. What is the underlying message Pablo Rodriguez is attempting to communicate to his daughter?
   a. He is too tired to attend her wedding.
   b. The enema has made him feel better.
   c. He is ready to give in to the disease and die.
   d. The enema has caused him pain.

12. Does the response by Pablo Rodriguez's daughter indicate a readiness to accept her father's condition?

13. _____ Pablo Rodriguez will be allowed to make the decision to forego further treatment without the approval of his immediate family. (True or False)

14. Identify referrals that may be beneficial for Pablo Rodriguez and his family at this time.

Care and Treatment of the Patient with Cancer

Reading Assignment: Care of the Patient with Cancer (Chapter 17)

Patient: Pablo Rodriguez, Room 405

Objectives:

1. Identify the physiological changes associated with the diagnosis of cancer.
2. List risk factors for the development of cancer.
3. Identify the tests that may be used to diagnose cancer.
4. Define metastasis.

Exercise 1

Writing Activity

 30 minutes

1. Which of the following foods have been shown to reduce the risk for cancer? Select all that apply.

   _____ Broccoli

   _____ Lettuce

   _____ Bananas

   _____ Carrots

   _____ Grapefruit

   _____ Tomatoes

2. Adding at least _____ servings of fruits and vegetables per day has been shown to reduce the risk for cancer.

3. _____ The risk for the development of lung cancer is similar among users of smokeless tobacco and cigarette smokers. (True or False)

4. Match each diagnostic test with its correct description. (*Hint:* See page 825 in your textbook.)

Diagnostic Test	Description
_____ Computed tomography	a. The use of noninvasive, high-frequency sound waves to examine external body structures.
_____ Radioisotope studies	
_____ Ultrasound testing	b. A computer is employed to process radio-frequency energy waves to assess spinal lesions, as well as cardiovascular and soft tissue abnormalities.
_____ Magnetic resonance imaging	
	c. The use or radiographs and computed scanning to provide images of structures at differing angles.
	d. A substance is injected or ingested; then the uptake is evaluated to identify areas of concern.

5. Which of the following characteristics are associated with benign growths? Select all that apply.

   _____ Rapid growth

   _____ Smooth and well-defined

   _____ Immobile when palpated

   _____ Often recurs after removal

   _____ Crowds normal tissue

   _____ Remains localized

6. Match each diagnostic laboratory test with the type of cancer it is used to detect. (*Hint:* See page 826 in your textbook.)

Diagnostic Test	**Type of Cancer Detected**
_____ Serum calcitonin levels	a. Thyroid, breast, and oat cell cancer in the lung
_____ Carcinoembryonic antigen	b. Gynecologic and pancreatic cancers
_____ PSA	c. Prostate cancer
_____ CA-125	d. Colorectal cancer

7. The complete blood cell profile of a patient diagnosed with cancer shows a reduction in the number of circulating platelets. Which of the following terms is used to describe this condition?
   a. Leukopenia
   b. Thrombocytopenia
   c. Anemia
   d. Neutropenia

8. Discuss the use of radiation treatments to manage cancer.

9. What is the mode of action for chemotherapy drugs?

10. Sometimes cancer is described as metastatic. What does this mean?

11. How does metastasis occur?

12. What diagnostic tools may be used to identify cancer? (*Hint:* See pages 824-826 in your textbook.)

13. Use of the immune system to counteract the destruction of cancer cells is known as

    _____. _____ may be used to remove a tumor, lesion, and surrounding malignant tissue.

14. Indicate whether each of the following statements is true or false.

    a. _____ Alopecia in patients undergoing chemotherapy results from damage to the hair follicle.

    b. _____ Alopecia is permanent.

    c. _____ Hair that regrows may be of a different color and/or texture than original hair.

15. List and discuss the complications involving the gastrointestinal system associated with the administration of chemotherapy.

16. Why is the patient with cancer at risk for developing nutritional problems?

17. For what nutritional disturbances is the patient with cancer at risk?

Exercise 2

 CD-ROM Activity

 30 minutes

- Sign in to work at Pacific View Regional Hospital for Period of Care 4. (*Note:* If you are already in the virtual hospital from a previous exercise, click on **Leave the Floor** and **Restart the Program** to get to the sign-in window.)
- From the Patient List, select Pablo Rodriguez (Room 405).
- Click on **Get Report** and read the Clinical Report.
- Click on **Go to Nurses' Station** and then on **Chart**.
- Click on **405** to view Pablo Rodriguez's chart.
- Click the **Nursing Admission** tab and review the information given.

1. What is Pablo Rodriguez's medical diagnosis?

2. According to the Nursing Admission, how does the patient describe his prognosis?

3. When was Pablo Rodriguez diagnosed with lung cancer?

→ • Click the **History and Physical** tab and review the reports.

4. How has Pablo Rodriguez's cancer been treated?

5. Does he have any family history of cancer?

6. Does his social history contain any risk factors for his diagnosis of lung cancer?

7. What psychosocial changes have resulted in his life because of the cancer?

8. Discuss the physical changes that have taken place as a result of Pablo Rodriguez's cancer.

9. Discuss Pablo Rodriguez's emotional readiness for death.

10. What emotional concerns have been voiced by the patient?

11. What therapeutic behaviors by the nurse are essential at this time?

12. What factors may put Pablo Rodriguez at risk for infection?

13. In addition to the nausea and vomiting, is Pablo Rodriguez suffering from any other complications of the gastrointestinal system?

14. Has Pablo Rodriguez experienced any nutritional disturbances during his illness?

LESSON **13** ────────────────────────

Assessment of the Patient with Gastrointestinal Complications

────────────────────────────────

✍ **Reading Assignment:** Care of the Patient with Gastrointestinal Complications
(Chapter 5)

Patient: Piya Jordan, Room 403

Objectives:

1. Identify clinical manifestations and causes of intestinal obstructions.
2. Develop nursing diagnoses appropriate for the patient experiencing an intestinal obstruction.
3. Explain operative measures used in cases of intestinal obstruction.
4. Identify common gastrointestinal disorders.
5. Identify tests used in the diagnosis of gastrointestinal disorders.
6. List medications used in the management of gastrointestinal disorders.

Exercise 1

 Writing Activity

 15 minutes

1. Describe the two types of intestinal obstructions.

   a. Mechanical obstruction:

   b. Nonmechanical obstruction:

2. The signs and symptoms associated with a bowel obstruction will be determined by the

   _____ and _____ of _____.

3. Early manifestations of an intestinal obstruction include which of the following? Select all that apply.

   _____ Loud bowel sounds

   _____ High-pitched bowel sounds

   _____ Vomiting

   _____ Constipation

   _____ Absence of bowel sounds

   _____ Frequent bowel sounds

   _____ Abdominal pain

 4. Identify several causes of mechanical intestinal obstructions. (*Hint:* See page 240 in your textbook.)

5. Which of the following are causes associated with non-mechanical intestinal obstructions? Select all that apply.

_____   Complications from surgery

_____   Bowel tumors

_____   Electrolyte abnormalities

_____   Thoracic spinal trauma

_____   Lumbar spinal trauma

_____   Emboli or atherosclerosis of the mesenteric arteries

_____   Impacted feces

6. _____   Paralytic ileus is the most common type of nonmechanical intestinal obstruction. (True or False)

7. What symptoms, if present, can be associated with a paralytic ileus?

_____   Increased abdominal girth

_____   Distention

_____   Urinary frequency

_____   Elevated white blood cell count

_____   Vomiting

8. What interventions are done to reduce the risk for developing a paralytic ileus?

_____   Abdominal assessment

_____   IV therapy

_____   Maintenance of NG tube

_____   Increase in patient activity

_____   Deep breathing exercises

Exercise 2

Writing Activity

 30 minutes

1. Match each diagnostic test with its correct description.

Diagnostic Test	**Description**
_____ Upper gastrointestinal study	a. Aspiration and review of stomach contents to determine acid production
_____ Tube gastric analysis	
_____ Esophagogastroduodenoscopy	b. Radiographs of the lower esophagus, stomach, and duodenum using barium sulfate at a contrast medium
_____ Lower GI endoscopy	c. Visualization of the upper GI tract by a flexible scope
_____ Bernstein test	
	d. An acid-perfusion test using hydrochloric acid
	e. Assessment of the lower GI tract with a scope

2. What is a KUB?

3. When providing education to a patient diagnosed with GERD, which of the following will need to be included in the teaching session? Select all that apply.

_____ Eat a low-fat, low-protein diet

_____ Avoid eating 4 to 6 hours before bedtime

_____ Remain upright for 1 to 2 hours after meals

_____ Avoid eating in bed

_____ Eat 4 to 6 small meals per day

_____ Reduce caffeine intake

4. Match each gastrointestinal disorder with its correct description.

Gastrointestinal Disorder

_____ GERD

_____ Candidiasis

_____ Gastritis

_____ Irritable bowel syndrome

_____ Ulcerative colitis

_____ Crohn disease

_____ Diverticulosis

Description

a. The presence of pouchlike herniations through the muscular layers of the colon

b. Characterized by inflammation of segments of the GI tract, resulting in a cobblestone-- like appearance of the mucosa

c. Episodic bowel dysfunction characterized by intestinal pain, disturbed defecation, or abdominal distention

d. The formation of tiny abscesses on mucosa and submucosa of the colon, producing drainage and sloughing of the mucosa and subsequent ulcerations

e. The backward flow of stomach acid into the esophagus

f. A fungal infection presenting as white patches on the mucous membranes

g. Inflammation of the lining of the stomach

5. Match each gastrointestinal medication with its correct classification.

Medication

_____ Maalox

_____ Pepcid

_____ Prevacid

_____ Carafate

_____ Cytotec

Classification

a. Proton pump inhibitor

b. Antacid

c. Antisecretory and cytoprotective agent

d. Mucosal healing agent

e. Histamine H_2 receptor blocker

6. Which of the following alternative therapies may provide relief for excessive flatulence? Select all that apply.

_____ Comfrey

_____ Queen Anne's lace seeds

_____ Anise

_____ Chaparral

_____ Peppermint oil

_____ Spearmint extract

7. Gastrointestinal disorders may be more prevalent in certain ethnic groups. Which of the following ethnic groups has a higher incidence of inflammatory bowel disease?
   a. Caucasian
   b. African-American
   c. Asian-American
   d. Americans of Middle Eastern descent

8. The increased incidence of gastritis in older adults can be attributed to the decreased secretion of _____.

9. What is a colectomy? What is a colostomy?

Exercise 3

 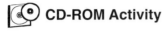 **CD-ROM Activity**

15 minutes

- Sign in to work at Pacific View Regional Hospital for Period of Care 1. (*Note:* If you are already in the virtual hospital from a previous exercise, click on **Leave the Floor** and then **Restart the Program** to get to the sign-in window.)
- From the Patient List, select Piya Jordan (Room 403).
- Click on **Get Report** and read the Clinical Report.
- Click on **Go to Nurse's Station** and then **403** to view Piya Jordan's chart.
- Click the **Emergency Department** tab and review the information given.

1. What are Piya Jordan's primary complaints upon arrival to the emergency department?

2. What are Piya Jordan's vital signs at admission?

   HR:

   T:

   RR:

   BP:

3. Piya Jordan's hypotension can most likely be attributed to which of the following?
   a. The presence of infection
   b. An elevation in blood glucose values
   c. Hypokalemia
   d. Dehydration

4. What diagnostic tests were ordered in the emergency department?

5. According to the ED Physician's Progress Notes, what are the abnormal findings on the physical assessment that support a potential bowel obstruction?

6. What are the treatment goals of the care for a patient experiencing an intestinal obstruction?

7. Initial management of the patient's condition included the placement of an NG tube. The NG tube can serve a variety of functions. Match each function with its correct description.

Function	Description
_____ Decompression	a. Irrigation of the stomach, used in cases of active bleeding, poisoning, or gastric dilation
_____ Feeding	b. Removal of secretions and gases from the GI tract
_____ Compression	c. Internal application of pressure by means of an inflated balloon to prevent internal GI hemorrhage
_____ Lavage	d. Installation of liquid supplements into the stomach

8. Piya Jordan has had the NG tube inserted for _____.

→ • Click **Return to Nurses' Station** and then **403** to go to Piya Jordan's room.
   • Review the **Initial Observations**.

9. According to the Initial Observations, blood is being administered to Piya Jordan. What laboratory results will necessitate close observation to determine the effectiveness of this intervention?

10. What will the nurse need to monitor concerning the blood transfusion?

11. Piya Jordan has remained NPO since the surgery. What information will the nurse need to monitor to ensure she is adequately hydrated?

Colorectal Cancer and Care of the Patient After Gastrointestinal Surgery

Reading Assignment: Care of the Surgical Patient (Chapter 2)
Care of the Patient with a Gastrointestinal Disorder (Chapter 5)

Patient: Piya Jordan, Room 403

Objectives:

1. Identify risk factors associated with the development of colorectal cancer.
2. List the warning signs and symptoms associated with a diagnosis of colorectal cancer.
3. Identify the assessment priorities for the postoperative patient.
4. Discuss the safe use of narcotics administered in the postoperative period.
5. Discuss the potential for postoperative complications.

Exercise 1

 Writing Activity

15 minutes

1. Indicate whether each of the following statements is true or false.

   a. _____ Cancer of the colon and rectum is the second leading cause of cancer in the United States.

   b. _____ In the early stages, colorectal cancer is often asymptomatic.

2. Match each location for colorectal cancer with its frequency of incidence. (*Hint:* See page 242 in your textbook.)

Location of Cancer	Frequency of Incidence
_____ Transverse splenic flexure, hepatic flexure, and descending colon	a. 45%
_____ Sigmoid and rectal	b. 25%
_____ Cecum and descending colon	c. 30%

3. The incidence of colorectal cancer is associated with which of the following? Select all that apply.

   _____ Ulcerative colitis

   _____ Peritonitis

   _____ Diverticulosis

   _____ Elevated bacterial counts in the colon

   _____ Vegan diets

   _____ High dietary fat intake

   _____ Dietary intake high in cruciferous vegetables

4. A patient at age 36 with a family history of colon cancer should follow which of the following recommendations for screening?
   a. Begin colonoscopy screening after age 50.
   b. Participate in a baseline colonoscopy prior to age 50.
   c. An initial colonoscopy should be performed prior to age 40 and repeated every 5 years.
   d. No special screening recommendations are needed.

5. Which of the following symptoms are associated with the later stages of colorectal cancer? Select all that apply.

   _____ Constipation

   _____ Diarrhea

   _____ Abdominal pain

   _____ Anemia

   _____ Weakness

   _____ Emaciation

6. The incidence of colorectal cancer increases in persons over age _____.

7. The 5-year survival rate for early localized colorectal cancer is _____%; for cancer that has spread to adjacent organs and lymph nodes, it is _____%.

8. _____ refers to weakness and emaciation associated with general ill health and malnutrition.

9. What details should be included in the assessment of a surgical incision?

Exercise 2

 CD-ROM Activity

 30 minutes

- Sign in to work at Pacific View Regional Hospital for Period of Care 1. (*Note:* If you are already in the virtual hospital from a previous exercise, click on **Leave the Floor** and **Restart the Program** to get to the sign-in window.)
- From the Patient List, select Piya Jordan (Room 403).
- Click on **Get Report** and read the Clinical Report.
- Click on **Go to Nurses' Station** and then click the **Drug** icon. Find the entry for meperidine and review.

1. Based on your review of the shift report, which care factors appear to be of high priority?

2. The assessment findings of which of the patient's body systems demonstrate the potential for developing postoperative complications?
   a. Respiratory system
   b. Renal system
   c. Integumentary system
   d. Reproductive system

- Click **Return to Nurses' Station**.
- Click on **403** and read the **Initial Observations**.
- Click on **Take Vital Signs** and then on **Clinical Alerts** and review the information given.
- Click **Patient Care** and complete a head-to-toe assessment.

3. Discuss the proper assessment of bowel sounds for this patient.

4. What is the purpose of the Jackson-Pratt drain? How long will it need to be in place for Piya Jordan?

5. When providing care for Piya Jordan, what should the nurse monitor and record regarding the NG tube?

6. Piya Jordan has a reduced aeration to the left lower lobe. What interventions can promote improved aeration and a reduction in potential complications?

→ • Click **Chart** and then **403** to view Piya Jordan's chart.
   • Click the **Nurse's Notes** tab and review the information given.

7. According to the Wednesday 0630 Nurse's Notes, Piya Jordan's meperidine PCA was discontinued because of suspicions of toxicity. Which of the following clinical manifestations are associated with meperidine toxicity? Select all that apply.

_____ Respiratory depression

_____ Systolic hypertension

_____ Clammy skin

_____ Cyanosis

_____ Stupor

_____ Coma

_____ Diarrhea

8. In the event that pharmacologic intervention is needed to treat meperidine toxicity, which of the following medications may be administered?
   a. Compazine
   b. Phenergan
   c. Morphine
   d. Narcan
   e. Famotidine

9. Which of the following conditions may increase a patient's risk for meperidine toxicity? Select all that apply.

_____ Advancing age

_____ Diabetes

_____ Cardiovascular disorders

_____ Renal impairments

_____ Hypertension

→ • Click **Physical Assessment** and complete a head-to-toe assessment.

10. Which of the following assessment findings for Piya Jordan are in accordance with the suspected meperidine toxicity? Select all that apply.

_____ Glasgow Coma Scale results

_____ Confusion

_____ Temperature 99.9

_____ Respiratory rate 23

_____ Slurred, slowed speech

_____ Restless

• Click **Return to Room 403**.
- Click **Patient Care** and then **Nurse-Client Interactions**.
- Select and view the video titled **0735: Pain—Adverse Drug Event**. (*Note:* If this video is not available, check the virtual clock to see if enough time has elapsed. The video cannot be viewed before its specified time.)

11. What problems were encountered during the previous evening with regard to the use of the PCA pump?

12. What patient/family concerns during the video indicate the need for education?

13. What issues does the nurse need to address with Piya Jordan's daughter in particular?

Exercise 3

 CD-ROM Activity

 30 minutes

- Sign in to work at Pacific View Regional Hospital for Period of Care 3. (*Note:* If you are already in the virtual hospital from a previous exercise, click on **Leave the Floor** and then **Restart the Program** to get to the sign-in window.)
- From the Patient List, select Piya Jordan (Room 403).
- Click **Get Report** and read the **Clinical Report**.
- Click **Go to Nurses' Station** and then **403** to enter the patient's room.
- Read the **Initial Observations**.

1. Have there been any changes in mental status since Period of Care 1?

2. What changes have been made to the type and/or administration of Piya Jordan's pain medication?

3. How does Piya Jordan rate her pain at this time?

 - Click **Chart** and then **403** to view Piya Jordan's chart.
- Click the **Surgical Reports** tab and review the reports.

4. What type of surgery was planned for Piya Jordan? What surgical procedure was actually completed?

5. Which of the following are the most common complications associated with the surgery performed on Piya Jordan? Select all that apply.

_____ Hemorrhage

_____ Infection

_____ Blood loss

_____ Pneumonia

_____ Wound dehiscence

_____ Blood clots

_____ Paralytic ileus

6. What is Piya Jordan's postoperative diagnosis?

➤ • Click the **Physician's Orders** tab and review the information given.

7. What medications and/or interventions have been ordered to assess and reduce the patient's postoperative risk of infection?

8. Which of the following assessments will provide information to determine the presence of an infection? Select all that apply.

_____ Vital signs

_____ Appearance of urine in Foley catheter bag

_____ Abdominal incision

_____ Lung fields

_____ Patency of Jackson-Pratt drain

➤ • Click **Return to Room 403**.
 • Click **Take Vital Signs** and review the information given.
 • Click **Patient Care** and perform a head-to-toe assessment.

9. Does Piya Jordan demonstrate any symptoms associated with a potential infection?

10. What interventions have been ordered to reduce the patient's risk for pulmonary complications?

Notes:

Notes:

Notes: